What Others Are Saying About This Book

A rich, informative, and moving collection of personal accounts, poems, and essays about the experiences caregivers face coping with Alzheimer's disease. I recommend caregivers read a few stories a day to help them better understand the disease, learn caregiving tips, and most of all realize that they are not alone.

David Troxel, MPH
Author, *The Best Friends Approach to Alzheimer's Care*
Alzheimer's Association—California Central Coast

With a touch of tears and sparkling humor, this book embraces caregivers' dedicated love and reinforces my need to care for my bride of fifty-two years as she cared for me.

Major Richard Jimmink, USAF Ret. & Caregiver

A   n-
ilies,   nd
other

                                                                    or
                                                                    n

T   n,
howe   by
descr

                                                                    ly
                                                                    er

T   d-
ness,   r-
stand   of
Alzh   ry
of m   n
from

                                                                    n
                                                                    th

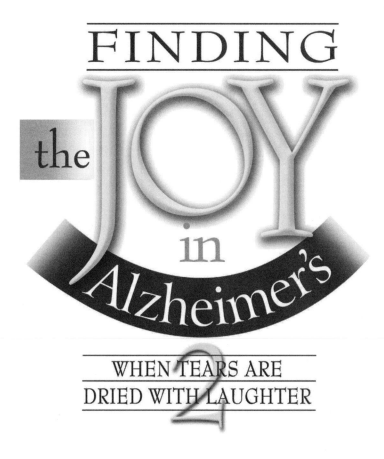

FINDING the JOY in Alzheimer's

WHEN TEARS ARE DRIED WITH LAUGHTER 2

BRENDA AVADIAN, M.A.

Author of *"Where's my shoes?" My Father's Walk Through Alzheimer's* and *Finding the JOY in Alzheimer's ~ Vol. I*

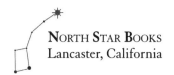

NORTH STAR BOOKS
Lancaster, California

We acknowledge the contributors for permission to include their material. (Contributions by the editor, Brenda Avadian, M.A., are not included in this listing.)

We have tried to learn the sources of the anonymous contributions sent via the Internet. If you can prove you are the original author/publisher of these Internet contributions, please contact North Star Books immediately. We want to give you credit.

Our mission is to bring JOY to caregivers of people with Alzheimer's and to use the sales proceeds to support organizations that help people with Alzheimer's and their families.

Coke is a registered trademark of The Coca-Cola Company.

JELL-O is a registered trademark of Kraft Foods, Inc.

Scrabble is a registered trademark of the Milton Bradley Company, division of Hasbro, Inc., in the United States and Canada and of J.W. Spear & Sons PLC., a subsidiary of Mattel, in Great Britain and elsewhere in the world.

Copyright © 2003 by Brenda Avadian, M.A., Editor

Library of Congress Publisher's Cataloging-in-Publication Data
Avadian, Brenda, M.A.
    Finding the joy in Alzheimer's ~ 2: When tears are dried with laughter / Brenda Avadian, M.A. — Lancaster, CA : North Star Books, 2003.
        175 p.   ill.   22 cm.
        1. Health—Alzheimer's disease 2. Caregivers—Alzheimer's disease 3. Alzheimer's disease—Patients—Care 4. Alzheimer's disease—Patients—Family relationships 5. Avadian, Brenda. I. Title
        ISBN 0-9632752-3-2 Trade paperback
        Library of Congress Control Number 2003111005

First Printing

Printed in the United States of America

NORTH STAR BOOKS
P.O. Box 259
Lancaster, California 93584
Telephone: 661.945.7529
E-mail: NStarBks@aol.com

Dedicated to
all family and professional caregivers
who work tirelessly
to provide quality care
for our loved ones.

Warning - Disclaimer

This book was written to help caregivers find joyful moments during the caregiving journey. It is sold with the understanding that the publisher and author are not rendering legal, medical, or other professional advice. If legal, medical, or other expert assistance is required, the reader should seek the services of a competent professional.

The named contributors retain the copyright to their material. They have signed a *Permission and Nonexclusive Rights Agreement* with the editor and publisher representing that they are the owner and creator of their submission(s) and give the editor and North Star Books permission to use the contribution(s).

The editor and North Star Books shall not have liability nor responsibility to any person and/or entity with respect to any loss or damage caused, or alleged to be caused, directly or indirectly by the information contained in this book.

If you do not wish to be bound by the above, you may return this book (in resalable condition) to the publisher for a refund.

Contents

SECTION FIVE: NEARING LIFE'S ULTIMATE TRANSITION

Acknowledgments

As with any undertaking, success rests not with the name on the cover but with everyone who selflessly offered their talents in order to complete this project. There are many who came forward to help. I thank each of them, because without them this book would not be.

First, and most important, are those people who shared their caregiving moments. To learn more about these contributors you may read their biographies at the end of this book.

Next are the members of our two-stage review teams who read and rated the submissions, and offered comments. Their job was difficult, yet I believe each person's opinion counted for a thousand others' and am pleased we had a demographically diverse review team. The reviewers include three contributors to Volume I, who also have stories in this book— Debbie Center, Linda Tucker, and Loraine Yates (they did not rate their own submissions)—my husband, David Borden; Dick Jimmink; June Cerza Kolf; and Jonathan Schulkin.

Third, I thank my longtime editor and text designer, Mary Jo Zazueta, who uses her magnifying glass to ensure what follows not only looks good but reads well; and my designer, Julia Ryan, who makes the best-designed Christmas cookies when she's not busy creating award-winning covers.

I extend *Special Thanks* to: Linda Tucker, Debbie Center, Sally Howard, and Kevin Fisher. Linda was available to answer my cries for help; Debbie created our subtitle; and Sally, my adopted mom, helped me with the administrative details (e.g., setting up a database and getting permissions).

Kevin worked miracles on the Internet whenever we had a crisis.

Finally, another huge thank-you to David Borden, my husband, who goes to work each day to support me while nearly everyone else I've mentioned joins me in touching the world's caregivers one book and one audience at a time.

Introduction

Is there JOY in Alzheimer's? In a word, YES! Caregivers are increasingly able to find the joyful side of Alzheimer's disease—that special moment when a loved one suddenly becomes aware and calls your name; a flash of innocence and childlike curiosity about something simple, like an ant on a picnic table; or the delight of clutching a favorite stuffed animal.

Caregivers often have life-changing experiences as they care for their loved ones. Both family and professional caregivers see firsthand that life is temporary. This reality spurs some caregivers to venture out to try new things, to strengthen their resolve to face the daily challenges of life, to try a new career or hobby, and even to write something for this volume. To renew themselves so that they can continue to care for their loved ones, some plan creative respites. One group of Internet chat room participants from diverse geographic locations gathers biannually in a selected city to raise funds for Alzheimer's while engaging in fun activities. Another caregiver finds respite at 13,500 feet!

When people first read the title, *Finding the JOY in Alzheimer's*, they pause, ponder, and then inquire or argue how we could suggest such a thing. In any case, this title is getting attention and inviting dialogue about a terminal disease that the media often presents as hopeless and depressing.

Alzheimer's is a serious disease that strikes an estimated eighteen million people worldwide, according to the World Health Organization.

Caring for a loved one with dementia caused by Alzheimer's is no laughing matter. Yet, caregivers are learning how to find some joy, no matter how small or great.

This second volume of *Finding the JOY in Alzheimer's: When Tears are Dried by Laughter* is a collection of candid stories written by the caregivers themselves, for the purpose of drying your tears of pain and fatigue with bursts of laughter. Amidst the clouds and thunderstorms of Alzheimer's, caregivers and their loved ones endure the rain and learn to relish each ray of sunshine. If for only a moment, this is what *Finding the JOY* is all about.

Take a moment for yourself right now and open this book. Gain comfort from reading other caregivers' stories and in knowing that we walk this road together. May these pages dry your tears with laughter and bring you enough strength to face today. Take a moment to read one story or poem daily. When you're finished, read the "Five Tips for Caregivers." Place your bookmark there and review the tips each time you feel the stress of caregiving.

My hope is that soon you will be *Finding the JOY in Alzheimer's*. Who knows? The third volume may include your experiences!

Finding the JOY in Alzheimer's ~ 2

SECTION ONE

CAREGIVERS

*D*eciding to care for a loved one is not easy. There are so many issues to consider—and there are many things that you can't even anticipate.

Years ago, my father's attorney listened as I complained about all the additional unexpected responsibilities of caring for my father. After making sense of my father's scrawled notes on scraps of paper tucked within the pages of a one-and-a-half-foot pile of newspapers, we discovered a bank account. We found a series of U.S. Savings Bond serial numbers written on index cards and various pieces of paper. David, my husband, painstakingly entered several hundred serial numbers into a file to send to the U.S. Department of Treasury, only to learn that many had been cashed in years earlier. It was endless. Each time we thought we were finished there was another piece of paper with information that we had to investigate.

David and I did not mind caring for my father as much as we disliked taking care of his estate and all the dreaded paperwork, plus dealing with my siblings.

The attorney said he understood my frustration and then painted a picture for me. "Brenda, when you decided to care for your father, you reached down to pick up a grain of sand; and you ended up with the whole beach!"

The telephone fell silent as I gulped, digested his words, and began to feel relief now that someone had placed our responsibilities into perspective.

Even after my father's passing in March 2001, the attorney's remark remains fresh in my mind.

If the estimated 50 million caregivers in the United States (according to a report by the National Family Caregivers Association) is any indication, there could be more than 100 million caregivers worldwide. These are significant figures and we need to give serious attention to these heroes who quietly provide billions of dollars worth of care.

Family and friends continue to carry the greatest weight. Many provide 7-day-a-week, 24-hour-a-day care for months or years; some continue providing care for decades. This comes at a price to the caregiver, to the family, to society, and ultimately to the world. What can we do to help?

Through projects like the *Finding the JOY* series, we are helping to educate the world about what it means to care for someone with Alzheimer's. We also need more programs to directly support the caregiver and to educate family members, and even nurses and doctors. How many times have we heard about a misdiagnosis ("He's just getting old.") or the unreasonable expectations of our loved ones with Alzheimer's?

As family caregivers walk this journey with their loved ones, they cope by attending support groups or participating in online chat rooms. Others try to schedule a respite, use the services of an adult day care center, or hire in-home healthcare. Yet, there are caregivers who cannot take advantage of needed services due to cost, lack of availability in their area, or no time to get away.

Even professional caregivers (those who receive pay) feel the burden. Many are responsible for more people than they can reasonably manage day after day. Imagine your loved one being one of eight, or even twelve, residents who receives maybe thirty to forty minutes of attention during an eight-hour shift from one harried nursing assistant who is also required to keep up with the daily paperwork. Is this any way to provide care for our loved ones?

Most professional caregivers are no less committed to providing quality care than are family members. Some grow close to our loved ones. Two Certified Nursing Assistants became so attached to my father they carried photos of him in specially made key fobs and charms. What a touching tribute, not to mention the feeling of comfort I had knowing how much they cared for my father.

As you hear the voices and read their stories and poems, we hope to touch all caregivers who feel alone and uncertain. We will continue to raise awareness in order to get the support these heroes deserve.

Meanwhile, let's walk this caregiving road together.

Superheroes

Caregivers are a unique group of people. What sets them apart is their resourcefulness in time of need, stamina in time of exhaustion, strength in time of weakness, and perseverance in time of futility. This makes caregivers sound like super-heroes.

Mary C. Fridley RN, C
Annapolis, Maryland

I Have AAADD!

I have recently been diagnosed with AAADD—Age Activated Attention Deficit Disorder!

This is why.

I decide to wash the car. I start toward the garage and notice the mail on the table. Okay, I'm going to wash the car, but first I'm going to go through the mail. I lay down the car keys on the desk, discard the junk mail, and I notice the trash-can is full.

Okay, I'll just put the bills on my desk and take the trash-can out, but since I'm going to be near the mailbox anyway, I'll pay these few bills first.

Now, where is my checkbook? Oops . . . there's only one check left. My extra checks are in my desk.

Oh, there's the Coke® I was drinking. I'm going to look for those checks. But first I need to put my Coke® further away from the computer. Oh maybe I'll pop it into the fridge to keep it cold for a while.

I head towards the kitchen and my flowers catch my eye. They need some water. I set down the Coke® on the counter and uh-oh, there are my glasses. I was looking for them all morning! I'd better put them away first.

I fill a container with water and head for the flowerpots—aaaarrgh!

Someone left the TV remote in the kitchen. We'll never think to look in the kitchen tonight when we want to watch television so I'd better put it back in the family room where it belongs.

I splash some water into the pots and onto the floor. I throw the remote onto a soft cushion on the sofa and I head back down the hall trying to figure out what it was I was going to do.

End of the day: The car isn't washed. The bills are unpaid. The Coke® is sitting on the kitchen counter. The flowers are half watered. The checkbook only has one check in it and I can't seem to find my car keys!

When I try to figure out why nothing was accomplished today, I'm baffled because: I KNOW I WAS BUSY ALL DAY LONG!!! I realize this is a serious condition and I'd get help—BUT FIRST, I think I'll check my e-mail . . .

Anonymous

What Makes Caregiving Rewarding?

As a young child, I would run to my mother to complain that once again I was a victim of some new injustice. She would hug me and wipe away my tears. The pain was gone. She always comforted me with the same advice. "Now don't worry, darling. This is good for your character!" My character? What did that mean?

After fifty years of marriage to a wonderful man and forty-five years of mothering four sons, I thought my character had been improved just about as much as it could be. Wrong. Wrong. Wrong.

Over ten years ago, when my husband, Sam, began to exhibit significant and persistent signs of memory loss, I didn't pay much attention. After all, I told myself, everyone is plagued with "senior moments" as they age. He too made light of his condition as he struggled valiantly to lead a normal life. But the process of his mental impairment was inexorable.

What a teacher he is! As my caregiving responsibilities increased, I came to understand and accept many lessons as blessings in disguise, blessings that were indeed "good for my character." I had experienced them previously, but not under such trying conditions.

Learning to be more patient—I, who was born under the bright star of Impatience, began moving more slowly, in harmony with his s-l-o-w rhythms.

Letting go of my stubborn need to be right. Ultimately, as I discovered, my being right makes absolutely no difference.

Enjoying humor as a great ally, a healing solvent for stress. Lightness often saves the day.

Learning how to better nourish myself emotionally and physically. When I ignore these basic needs, I am diminished in my caregiving ability.

And, the biggest lesson of all: Refusing to cling to the past. Remembering what was then only brings me anguish now.

Most of all I came to realize that caring for Sam is life itself—that nothing I can read or study—nothing I can talk about—is as important or real as simply being present with him right here, right now.

Each day brings its own blessings in disguise. And each day, in fantasy, I share with my mother what is going on. I imagine her hugging me. This time we embrace as woman to woman. She no longer advises what is "good for my character."

We just smile at each other.

Phyllis Major
Palm Desert, California

A Caregiver's Prayer

In the late night hours,
I lay my weary head.
Reaching for the monitor,
That sits beside my bed.

I listen for her breathing,
Or her little moans.
I hear her gentle whispers,
To someone she has known.

Then I lay me down to sleep,
And this is what I pray:
Lord, I ask for peace tonight,
And in her bed, she'll stay.

Give me strength to give the care,
That she truly needs.
Help me bring her comfort,
And in me, plant a seed.

One that blooms of Kindness,
With a fragrance of Your Grace.
Faith that You will guide me,
And Love that shines my face.

Help me with my patience,
And let my heart expand.
And if there's much confusion,
Lord, please . . . help her understand.

As we walk this journey,
Please keep us in Your sight.
Thanks so much for listening,
And we'll talk tomorrow night.

Loraine Yates
Ontario, California

Grounded at 13,500 Feet

As caregivers, I think one of the most important (and hardest) lessons to learn is to take time for ourselves. After many years of caring for my *Little Mama*, I'm finally learning! So, every two or three months I plan a short getaway. This is a little story of my February trip.

I decided that since I would be turning the BIG 5-0 this year I was going to plan something from my "Always wanted to do" list. With help from a dear friend, plans were set. I was going to go SKY DIVING! As my girlfriend said, I was going to be *falling* into fifty!

On February 8, 2002, at 1:45 p.m., I JUMPED from a plane at 13,500 feet! Caption: It was the most exhilarating experience of my life! It was awesome! For the next few weeks I was flying high —even at ground level! I couldn't wait to get home so my family could see the video that was made of my jump.

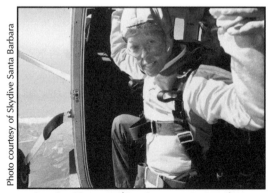

Photo courtesy of Skydive Santa Barbara

Loraine Yates ready to jump at 13,500 feet.

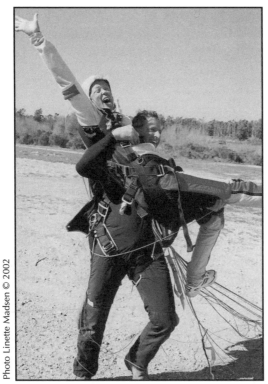

Photo Linette Madsen © 2002

After a successful jump, Loraine Yates is lifted off her feet by Stanley R. Olzaski, instructor at Skydive Santa Barbara.

The night after I returned home, my husband, my eighty-seven-year-old *Little Mama*, and I gathered in the den for the big show. I told Mama she was going to see what I had done while I was gone and how I had celebrated my fiftieth birthday.

She seemed excited, and I was still flying high!

As the tape began and the title *Skydive Santa Barbara* came up I looked over at her and saw a very worried look on her face. Tears were welling up in her eyes and my heart sank. I asked her what was wrong and she said she was scared. I tried to tell her there was nothing to be worried about, that I was here. I was safe and sound and I was sorry this upset her.

She turned to my husband, Larry, and asked him if he knew I was going to do this and how could he allow me to do this?

Larry and I laughed and he told her he had absolutely NO say in the matter!

As the tape continued, she kept saying, "I can't believe it! I just can't believe this!"

Since it was upsetting Mama, I decided to stop the tape. Larry and I would view the rest of it upstairs.

My *Little Mama* took my hand and asked if I had any more trips planned. I replied, "No."

As she turned to leave the room, she said, "Good! Because you can't *ever* go away again. You are on RESTRICTION!"

As Larry and I retired upstairs, I thought, Boy, my little celebration party didn't go very well! Little did I know that I would be put on restriction at fifty and grounded at 13,500 feet!

This is a getaway I will never forget!

Loraine Yates
Ontario, California

SECTION TWO

LESSONS FROM OUR LOVED ONES

*A*n inspiring story made the rounds on the Internet about an elderly woman, whose husband of seventy years died. After his death she had to be placed in a nursing home. Despite being blind, she was well-poised and fashionably dressed with makeup and coiffed hair. She was a most-appreciative, gracious, and dignified lady.

When she arrived at the nursing home, her room was not ready, so she waited in the lobby for a few hours. When the room was finally ready and her paperwork complete, she listened as her friend began describing in detail how the room was decorated.

Before her friend could finish, the lady interrupted her and said, "I love it." She insisted that "seeing" the room had nothing to do with what she felt in her heart. She explained that *happiness* is a decision everyone makes in advance. She had made the decision to like her room.

She added that every morning she can decide to either recount her pains and struggles or to be thankful for what she has and is able to do. She chooses to be thankful.

※ ※

Caregivers regularly make decisions on how they will get through each day, especially when they have to hurdle many obstacles (e.g., finances, family members, health care, and housing options). This lady teaches us that we have a choice about how we will cope with each day that we care for our loved ones.

※ ※

Nearly five million Americans, and an estimated eighteen million people worldwide, have Alzheimer's and walk this one-way road into darkness without being able to communicate in a meaningful way. The last stage of Alzheimer's often means that family and friends are long forgotten, communication is nil, and a caregiver is responsible for all of your needs.

As I faced my father's decline and as I witness the decline of dear friends today, I wonder what it would be like to walk to the end of this road, where I would require total care and be unable to communicate my thoughts or to be understood. Imagining this helps me feel the fear, the helplessness, and even the joy mixed with frustration.

For example, I like wearing turtlenecks during the day and having the blankets tucked under my chin and around my ears at night so that my neck stays warm. But, my caregivers dress me in open-collared clothing that easily slips over my head and hangs loosely over my body, giving me the chills. I don't like the way they wash me in the shower. (Each of us has a unique way of cleaning our body. Some of us linger underneath the hot running water, while others get this business done in military fashion.) The water my caregivers use is not hot enough. While they're soaping me, they don't leave the warm water running over my body to keep me warm. I get chilled when they dry me.

As I continue to imagine what it is like to live with dementia, I wonder, Will my caregivers be patient with me? Will they remember to talk into my right ear because I cannot hear with my left? Or when they talk in my left ear and I chuckle or awkwardly reply, will they simply attribute it to dementia? Will I be given a room with quiet roommates or loud ones who scream or are up all night? Will they involve me in activities and allow me to be alone when I want to be alone? (How will they know the difference if I cannot tell them?) Will they come when I need them, even if I don't know how to call them?

When I try to imagine all of this, I become afraid. Yet, I can better view the world in which our loved ones live, a world that is void of self-control. This is frightening when I honestly consider it. And I become humbled and filled with more compassion.

I appreciate the lucid moments that our loved ones experience—when they recognize us and say the right things. I listen with wonder when they speak about Mom and Dad, brother and sister, and dear friends who have long since departed. Sometimes they speak so vividly, I wonder if they have a special connection to the afterlife. I sit and enjoy the stories of their youth, whether real or fabricated. I imagine them when they were young, running around, playing, going to school, falling in love, having big dreams, marrying, and raising children. But, as quickly as lucidity arrives, it flees. And the silence returns.

Those who have Alzheimer's are no different than you or me. Many live the reality they knew some forty years earlier—they typically express concern for taking care of the children or going to work. They are among the best storytellers. It is no wonder that some adult day care programs pair the very young with our elderly loved ones. What a benefit to both—they enjoy each other's company and learn from one another. It's a great way for our loved ones to have a reason to live day-to-day and a wonderful place where children have a truly caring audience.

In truth, I can only guess how the brain suffers so much

damage that my father eventually forgot he was married (he married late in life, at age forty) and my whole existence was wiped clean from the increasingly blank slate of his mind. I don't know how spouses or life partners cope with losing their loved ones after fifty and sixty years of being together. What a loss.

It is in the midst of this ongoing loss that we grasp for the few rays of sunshine that break through the clouds of Alzheimer's, the warm light that brings us joy and dries our tears with laughter.

And, if we can learn something from our loved ones' journey; this is even better!

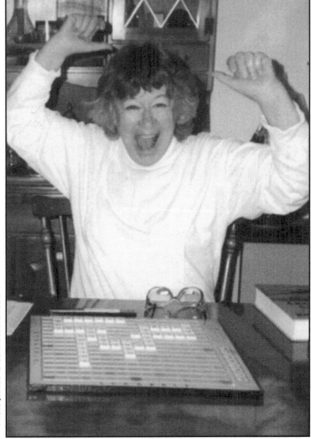

Photo Janice Greenhouse ©1996

Victory! Janette Shulman of Colorado may show signs of early Alzheimer's, but she hits yet another BINGO by using all seven letters in a game of Scrabble®.

The Power of a Smile

Our mom is eighty-six years old. When she lost her independence by giving up driving two years ago, she moved in with my sister, Linda, in Lancaster, California. Shortly thereafter, Mom started showing noticeable signs of Alzheimer's.

Linda's e-mail brought a smile to my face: *I came home from work and was puzzled to find all of my dirty dishes on the kitchen counter. I opened the dishwasher to find that our family's dirty socks had been carefully arranged on the prongs inside and put through the dishwashing cycle. Thankfully, Mom didn't put the dishes in the washing machine.*

Before this, Mom had lived alone in a house I owned in Palmdale, California. She was extremely active in her church and stayed busy taking care of the house as well as writing to me and forwarding my mail. She said she was living vicariously through my letters that told of my husband's and my adventures as fulltime RVers. She was as excited about our travels as we were.

Eventually, though, Mom stopped writing to us. Instead, we started following Mom's progress with Alzheimer's through Linda's e-mail messages and phone calls. Some of Mom's experiences definitely brought chuckles.

Another e-mail from Linda: *The rolls of toilet paper and paper towels ran out at the same time. You can probably guess what I found upon returning home from work. The toilet paper was on the paper towel rack in the kitchen and the paper towels were standing by the toilet in the bathroom.*

While talking with Linda over the telephone, she told us something else that Mom did. *We had a lazy Susan dish on the counter with different snacks in each dish. When all the nuts in one dish were gone, Mom tried to help. She filled it with dry dog food.*

The hardest thing for Mom to remember was whether to use the liquid dish soap or the powdered dishwasher soap in the dishwasher. The first time she used liquid soap, Linda opened the dishwasher in mid-cycle to add a dirty glass. Suds poured out onto the floor.

While I was home for a visit, Mom unintentionally taught us an important lesson about a smile. When Linda would come into the room with a serious expression on her face, Mom wouldn't recognize her. In fact, Mom would ask her with much concern, "Where is Linda?" On the other hand, when Linda walked in with a smile, Mom would say, "Oh, hi, Linda. I am so glad to see you." Come to think of it, when Mom returns our smiles with her own lovely smile, it warms our hearts, too.

Barbara Jacobson
Livingston, Texas

Time Stood Still

"What is your biggest problem these days?" a friend recently asked me. I did not hesitate in replying that my biggest problem was my enemy: Time. Time moves too fast—seems like it moves faster than the speed of light. I've heard others express a similar thought, especially seniors like myself. How I'd love to slow it down.

A short while ago a wonderful thing happened to help me deal with time. My husband, Phil, and I live in a residential continuing care community. Phil has Alzheimer's but is able to reside with me in the independent living section. We were fortunate to be invited to join the residents of the Alzheimer's unit on a picnic in a nearby park.

We settled down at a picnic table by the edge of the lake with several other residents and began to enjoy our picnic lunch.

While we ate, these folks began to observe the wondrous forces of nature around us, with awe. They relished the ducks and geese that came close to our table, commenting on the different sounds. They looked out over the water and enjoyed seeing a sailboat slowly glide past, and they were fascinated by the speed of a motorboat. Looking in another direction, they noticed some kids in a small boat trying to catch fish.

There was a childlike wonder that unfolded and a joy that I cannot describe. Something touched them deeply—perhaps early childhood memories.

Even the food at the table was savored in a way I had long forgotten. When they observed an ant, they followed it with their eyes as if they had not seen one before.

I was nearly in tears. I will never forget the wondrous

looks on their faces. It didn't take long for me to feel transformed at this table where God was surely present.

My gift that day was twofold. One, to us, the quality of life for people with memory loss may seem to be gone, but there is joy present in their souls—a sense of wonder that can only be experienced in the present. Two, I came to realize the secret to making time slow down was to join their lovely world of wonder at all of God's creations.

Wherever we are, the beauty of God's creativity is around us, and can fill us with awe. It isn't always easy to take time to appreciate our surroundings. Yet, this gift is ours if we just take the time to use all of our senses. Then, a moment can seem like a lifetime. What a gift. Time is no longer the enemy when we cherish the present.

I will treasure forever that day in the park when time stood still.

Sharon Wright, Ed.D., MFT
LaVerne, California

Garden of Joy

Bright and sunny days of Spring
Or crisp days of Fall.
We walk together, hand in hand
The Good times we recall.

We stroll along the garden.
I take your fragile hand.
You love to feel the petals
And walk barefoot through the sand.

Oh, how you love the flowers
All shades of pink and red.
Smelling sweet the fragrance
As you slowly tip your head.

Together as we wander
Among the shared trees,
We speak of olden days
That bring back memories.

And as the days grow shorter
We'll spend the hours well.
I'll treasure every moment
For only time will tell.

How long 'til the angels call you
To make the journey Home.
All sorrows, we will leave behind
The Garden, we will roam.

And if there is a moment
When I am feeling sad.
I'll think back to the Garden
And the good times that we had….

Loraine Yates
Ontario, California

It Pays to Go to School

A couple of childhood sweethearts, who were married and lived in the same neighborhood they were raised in, celebrated their fiftieth wedding anniversary by visiting their old high school. They held hands as they found the desk they'd shared—the one on which he had carved "I love you, Dolores."

On their way home, they froze when they heard tires squeal as an armored truck tried to turn too fast around a corner. Suddenly, the back doors flung wide open and a bag of money fell out rolling to a stop right in front of their feet. Dolores quickly picked it up. They didn't know what to do with it, so they took it home.

At home, she counted the money—fifty thousand dollars. Her husband, Bob, exclaimed, "We've got to give it back!"

Confident in the law, she replied, "Finders keepers," and put the money back into the bag and hid it up in their attic.

The following day, two FBI agents walked door-to-door in the neighborhood asking each of the residents about the money. Dolores and Bob answered the door.

After introducing themselves, one of the FBI agents asked, "Did either of you see a bag of money that fell out of an armored truck yesterday?"

Dolores quickly replied, "No."

Bob corrected her and added, "She's lying. She hid it up in the attic."

Dolores explained, "Don't believe him, he has Alzheimer's."

The agents, thinking they may have found the money, invited Bob to sit down and tell his version of what happened. "Tell us the story from the beginning," one said.

43

Bob sat up and explained, "Well, when Dolores and I were walking home from school yesterday ...."

The FBI agent turned to see his partner's reaction. They both sighed and shook their heads. "Well, I think we're finished here."

Anonymous
Revised by Editor

Lobster and Hot Dogs

One day after visiting Edith, one of the residents who used to dine with my father at the nursing home, I walked over to the nurses' station. As the staff and I were updating one another about our activities one of the residents walked up to the window and stood quietly by my side. I noticed a remote control in her hand. I wondered how she had managed to get it and if the staff and residents in the activity room were looking for it.

I turned to her and said, "You must be in charge here."

"No, I'm not," she said, not turning her head, but still looking at the nursing staff.

"You sure?" I asked. "You've got the remote. That means you're in control."

Turning in my direction, she said, "Nope. Not in control."

For a moment I wondered if she was a resident, because she was responding quite well considering we were in the section where residents have late Alzheimer's. I paused, debating whether or not I should offer a teasing remark. Then I noticed that most of the staff members at the nurses' station were watching the two of us.

"Oh, you must be the supervisor, then." I was trying to get some clarification and turned to the staff members, who were now smiling.

"No, I'm not!" she insisted.

"Oh, I'm sorry," I said apologetically, "you're the manager?"

"If I were, I'd change things around here!" she said, sizing me up with her eyes.

Uh-oh, what have I started? I thought. But, being an instigator and knowing the staff would probably not want to hear what came next, I pursued this line of discussion while winking at the staff, "Oh? What would YOU change?" I asked.

"I'd fire the cook!"

The staff breathed a sigh of relief and chuckled that she was not blaming them for anything.

"Really, why?"

No answer. Oops, that question was too open-ended. She was unable to respond.

"Because they don't serve lobster and caviar?" I prompted. I was always teasing the cook, administrator, and the nursing staff about the need to serve lobster and caviar. Whenever residents waited for their food to arrive and would ask what they were eating that day I'd answer loudly, "LOBSTER and CAVIAR!" They always looked at me and then laughed.

She looked at me again, "Lobster . . ."

"Caviar?" I hinted.

"No."

She seemed to know what she wanted.

"Lobster," she repeated and paused. "Lobster . . . and hot dogs."

"Lobster and hot dogs?" I asked in surprise.

"Yes, lobster and hot dogs," she repeated with certainty.

I looked at the staff and we laughed. There was hope. Maybe we would see a change in the menu yet!

"I'll talk with the cook immediately and make sure these changes are made," I said.

Satisfied, she walked away.

The staff laughed and added, "Good luck!"

Brenda Avadian, M.A.
Lancaster, California

Food Fight by Candlelight

When my mother was diagnosed with Alzheimer's, I was fortunate to be able to place her in a nursing home about five minutes away from where I lived. This allowed me to visit with her at least several times a week. We took walks together, and before she was really sick, we would go out for dinner, lunch, or ice cream. She was an avid reader, and I took books to her all of the time. And, when she could no longer read, I would sit and read to her. I was fortunate to be able to spend a lot of time with Mom in the last years before her death.

After a while, Alzheimer's played the cruel trick of role reversal with Mom and me. There were times when she would call me *Mom*. She also started acting like a three-year-old in stressful situations. I was getting complaints from the home that she would hit other residents for no apparent reason. Before Alzheimer's struck, Mom was a sweet, kind, and quiet person.

Having Mom act like a three-year-old was quite a surprise for me, especially since she created havoc when we were together. In fact, there is one particular event that comes to mind.

The nursing home in which I placed Mom was quite nice. In addition to regular events and activities, they also hosted elegant dinners for residents and their guests. These were wonderful dinners with white tablecloths and linen napkins. The meal was served by candlelight and a pianist played music for everyone's enjoyment. They were lovely, elegant evenings, and Mom and I always looked forward to them.

At our last elegant dinner Mom was starting to show the

effects of the Alzheimer's. We were served a menu of baked, boneless chicken breast, mashed potatoes with butter, a vegetable, hot rolls, and wine, dessert, and coffee.

We sat at a table with another resident and her guest. During dinner Mom kept trying to eat her roll with a fork and her mashed potatoes with her hand. I cleaned the potatoes from her hand and gave her the fork. Then I broke her roll into small pieces. After my third attempt at encouraging Mom to use a fork for her mashed potatoes, she stabbed her roll with the fork, grabbed a handful of mashed potatoes, and threw the glob into my face.

Everyone who saw the food missile hit me gasped and then started to laugh. Soon all of us were laughing. The laughter made my mom laugh, too. All this laughter brought the nurses in to see what was happening.

As one of the nurses helped me clean up, I told her "I think this is the last of our candlelight dinners."

And, unfortunately, it was.

Shirley Jenkins
Anaheim, California

Write it Down!

A couple in their eighties were having problems remembering things, so they went to the doctor to see if anything was seriously wrong. They described their memory problems.

After examining the couple, the doctor said they were fine physically. He then advised them that one way to reduce their forgetfulness was to write things down.

The couple thanked the doctor and left.

Later that night while watching TV, the man got up from his chair and his wife asked, "Where are you going?"

"To the kitchen," he replied.

"Will you get me a bowl of ice cream?"

"Sure."

To be certain he'd remember, she asked, "Don't you think you should write it down?"

"No, I can remember."

"Well, okay. I would also like some strawberries on top," she said. "You'd better write that down, because I know you'll forget."

Slightly irritated, he insisted, "I can remember that you want a bowl of ice cream with strawberries."

Somewhat surprised, but still wanting to make sure he wrote it down, she added, "Well, I would also like whipped cream on top. You'd better write *that* down."

Now completely irritated at her insistence, he sternly clarified, "I don't need to write it down! I can remember it." Fuming, he walked into the kitchen.

About twenty minutes later he returned from the kitchen and handed her a plate of bacon and eggs. She stared at the plate for a moment and said angrily, "I TOLD you to write it down! You forgot my toast!"

Anonymous

I Developed Hemorrhoids!

While providing social services at a skilled nursing facility in Loma Linda, California, I witnessed a number of memorable interactions among residents, their family members, and our staff. But one incident stands out more than others. Although residents in nursing homes come from different economic and social levels, they are treated much the same by the staff. It is the responsibility of the social worker to provide information about the patient's life to the staff. This is especially important when the patient suffers from dementia, as he or she is unable to provide this information.

Staff, resident, and family had gathered for the convalescent facility's regular care plan meeting. Staff members were seated on one side of the long table, facing the resident, Mrs. Dickerson, and her daughter. Jill had a protective arm over her mother's shoulder in preparation for the beginning of the meeting.

I couldn't help but notice the contrast between the white uniforms of the nursing director and her staff, and the bright blue and orange hues of Jill's designer outfit. I am sure that I heard Jill's Gucci shoes rhythmically tapping the yellowed linoleum floor as she impatiently waited for the last staff person to arrive.

Mrs. Dickerson was one of those Alzheimer's patients that the staff refers to as "pleasantly confused." Mrs. Dickerson sat quietly at her daughter's side, dressed in her best senior citizen duster. It was evident that Mrs. Dickerson had recently visited the facility's beauty shop, probably in anticipation of her daughter's visit. A sweet, vacant smile played across her face.

Mrs. Dickerson remained quiet during the course of the meeting, which the nursing director chaired. Her daughter Jill was anything but quiet. She routinely questioned each assessment and answered any and all questions that were directed toward her mother. Finally, in desperation, the nursing director turned to our pleasantly confused resident, requesting some information regarding her life before entering the facility.

Jill eyed the nursing director seated across the table. It was obvious that she believed the nursing director was as dumb as dirt. Didn't she know that Alzheimer's patients couldn't remember?

With an air of disgust, Jill stated loudly to all the staff present, "You are wasting your time asking these questions of my mother. My mother doesn't remember anything about her life. She has no memory of her marriage, her children, or her high school years."

Upon hearing this pronouncement, Mrs. Dickerson sat up straight, assumed an air of authority, and rose from her chair. Looking around the room at the faces of the staff members and her daughter, she stated grandly, "That is not true." I remember my high school years vividly! That is when I developed hemorrhoids!" Mrs. Dickerson sat down with a flourish.

Roberta Wertenberg
Yucaipa, California

Screaming Lady

In July 1999, I finally had to place my husband, Don, in a secured skilled nursing home specializing in Alzheimer's care.

I visited him almost every day.

One day we were in the activity room and one of the residents was screaming. A few of the other residents told her to be quiet; in fact, their exact words were, "Shut up!"

She continued to scream, "Where's my husband?"

Tired of hearing her, one of the other residents said, "He's probably out with a lady who doesn't scream!"

The room roared with laughter.

This outburst quieted her for about five minutes.

Marion Riley
Lancaster, California

God's Wedding Day Confetti

I don't know what it's like to approach Alzheimer's gradually. Mom had virtually no recognizable symptoms one day—and the day following surgery she wasn't the same person.

The afternoon after Mom's knee replacement surgery, her nurse was waiting for me when I came to visit. She started explaining Sundown Syndrome. She was surprised when I said, "That's not anything new. I just didn't know what to call it. And, by the way, it doesn't only happen at sundown."

I learned later that anesthesia can cause dramatic changes and that it is common for this to happen with Alzheimer's patients. It was the first time anyone said *Alzheimer's disease*.

I didn't have a clue what Alzheimer's really was.

A week later the hospital discharged Mom to a rehab unit in the facility across the street. After three weeks she was fighting to come home but they said, "She is not ready to go home, physically or mentally." I knew she had regressed but I assumed getting her home would speed up recovery. I was convinced life would go back to the way it had been.

It took another week of assuring the rehab unit staff that Mom, Dad, and I lived together and that if Dad and I couldn't care for her, we would hire help as needed. They let Mom come home early. Mom improved, but life was never the same. I believe we were lucky—the sudden progression of symptoms was better then getting an early diagnosis and living with the fear of what was to come.

Five years later, at ninety-three, Mom sits in our home for long periods of time, staring vacantly. She dozes often.

Attempts at conversation with her are frustrating. Mom

doesn't know what to do and is constantly asking what she is supposed to do next.

For example, she can make it to the bathroom with her wheeled walker, but occasionally forgets to remove her clothing—and then it's too late. She remembers things from many years ago—but can't remember what I told her two minutes ago. Each time we have an incident that requires a trip to the hospital, the nurse will ask the usual orientation questions, and then give up when Mom can't tell her what *time* of day, let alone what *day* it is.

Although the start of the holidays seemed especially difficult this year, Christmas came and we had a good day with family and other visitors. The next day Mom began a downward spiral that continued through New Year's Day, when she lost continence. When she could put words together, they were caustic. She was hardly eating, not even her favorite: chocolate. She spent most of her time curled up under blankets. Dad and I believed she would not recover this time. We would no longer be able to handle the situation alone at home.

The next day Mom started to turn around. Every day seemed a little bit better. Life gradually was returning to normal for us. January was nearly gone; Mom and Dad's anniversary would be on the twenty-fifth.

※ ※

It snowed the night before Mom and Dad were married in 1948. The wedding party and guests had a difficult time getting to the church and the reception. The snow continued lightly all morning and the wedding pictures made the snowflakes look like confetti.

꙳ ꙳

This winter it was not nearly as cold and we would be able to get Mom out easily, but I was debating whether or not to bother having any celebration. After all, Mom wouldn't know the difference and Dad wouldn't care. I had second thoughts and did some quick preparations.

It had been a very confusing day for Mom—but we went out to dinner anyway. Surprisingly, many people we knew were at the restaurant. Quite a few came over to say hi. I quietly told them there would be cake later.

Dinner was uneventful. The chef made a wonderful scallop and shrimp entree with lobster sauce arranged over tiny, subtly spiced pasta pancakes. Mom asked several times if I had made sure the dogs were okay before we left, and there was other small talk.

We finished up with a huge chocolate cake frosted with sweetened whipped cream. Singing waitresses delivered it to the table. The whole room joined in the singing. Mom was searching around, trying to see where the cake was going. She was a little bewildered when it landed in front of her and Dad.

As people took a piece of cake, offered congratulations, and dispersed, Mom leaned over to ask me what the fuss was about.

"It's your anniversary," I said.

"Oh, is it?" she asked. "What is today's date?"

"January 25," I said.

She sat up a bit and said, "Oh, yeah it is!" and smiled.

On the way home Mom asked at least six times why there had been cake and a celebration. Then, suddenly recalling her snowy cold wedding day fifty-four years ago, she remarked, "But there is no confetti! It's too warm!" Then she laughed.

The story had always been that God supplied *real confetti* on their wedding day.

Denise E. Kelley
East Falmouth, Maine

A Million Accident-Free Miles

Like so many other middle-aged women, I didn't fully understand the devastating effects of Alzheimer's disease until my father was diagnosed with it. I'd read articles and personal stories dealing with this mind-stealing illness, but nothing prepared me for actually living with the gut-wrenching emotions Alzheimer's brings to a family.

The signs were subtle at first. Dad would completely forget what he was talking about in mid-sentence. Then it progressed into Dad getting lost going to the neighborhood grocery store. My brothers, sister, and I went about our busy lives figuring that if Mom wasn't too concerned about it, we shouldn't be either. After all, we reasoned, Dad was seventy. We had to accept the fact that he was getting old.

When Mom died after a brief illness we were forced to take notice of Dad's increasingly strange behavior, which was now out of control.

It's emotionally heartbreaking to become a parent to your own parent; to lose a father but gain a child, which is what happens when Alzheimer's comes into your life.

Dad had traveled a million *accident-free* miles throughout his career as a truck driver. An award for this proud accomplishment hung over his bed. It was now our responsibility to tell a man who had steered some of the largest semis around the city that he could no longer drive his car around the neighborhood. But, that's just what we had to do. I soon found myself relating to the helplessness other middle-aged children felt taking care of a parent whose mind was faltering.

Inevitably, the time came when we had no choice but to place Dad in a nursing home after he almost burned down the kitchen. We were faced with the stark reality that this was where he belonged—for his own safety as well as our sanity. I was just beginning to find out that making the transition to becoming my father's keeper would not be an easy one.

On that first day at the nursing home, I felt the same queasy feeling I had when my daughter began her first day of kindergarten. On that long ago day, I had wanted to hug her and take her back home with me. Instead, I hid my tears and encouraged her to join the rest of the kids at play. I found it just as emotional leaving Dad behind in the strange confines of the nursing home.

As an orderly attached electronic bracelets to Dad's wrists, I sadly realized that my father would never be free again— mentally or physically. It was hard watching Dad live out the rest of his life trapped in a living purgatory, not really here, not really gone.

Dad suffered with Alzheimer's for about six years before his death finally set him free. But truthfully, even though I lost my father, as I had known him, many years before his death, I was also fortunate to see a side of him I might never have experienced had it not been for Alzheimer's.

There were tender moments when he'd touch my cheek and call me by name. I'd feel so elated that he had recognized me, though I knew the moment would be fleeting. I was surprised to realize that this debilitating disease could teach me life's lessons. These sentiments wouldn't be lost on me anytime soon.

I remember seeing a man's integrity in action, even though the frail, delicate frame of an old man had replaced his once strong physique. I'd watch as Dad stood at the nurses' station inquiring about a job. "I can work," he'd tell anyone who would listen. He was never the type to take something for nothing, which is why he felt it so important to pay for his meals.

I noticed during my visits that most of the patients possessed the same admirable qualities as Dad. Honest, decent people who'd fought in wars and worked hard to give their families a better life. Young mommies who used to rock their little ones to sleep, now geriatric patients clutching soft dolls to their chests as they spent their last days reliving what meant the most to them a long time ago.

Though their thin bodies were broken and their minds faded, their loving gestures were a testament that some habits born of the heart can never be broken.

I have seen countless lonely souls strolling the endless hallways of nursing homes, waiting for the chance to connect with a warm smile, to feel the gentile touch of someone reaching out to hold their hand, or to hear a few kind words.

I've noticed that most of these older folks come alive with wide-eyed enthusiasm at the opportunity to retell stories of *the good old days*. Most cannot remember their children's names, but amazingly can recall their own childhoods as if they happened yesterday.

Dad managed to get out of the nursing home once, even though he still wore the magnetic bracelets that set off the exit alarms. He hailed a cab, and instructed the driver to take him to Canaryville, a Chicago community. He gave the address of his boyhood home, a place he'd lived more than sixty years ago.

I watched my dad grow old; his mind riddled with confusion. And yet, his soul lived in an era no disease could take away. I guess it just goes to show that no matter where the miles may take us, we always travel back to our childhood—that safe and secure place locked in our memories.

When I received the call my father was dying I felt both panic and relief. The middle-age part of me was happy that he was finally at peace—no more confusion, no more restless agitation. But there was the little girl in me who would miss the man who could make everything okay—a man whose strength would move mountains if his family needed him to.

As I sit here, with graying hair and multiplying wrinkles, I find contentment in my own childhood memories, of a dad who chased away monsters and calmed the fears that midnight storms would sometimes bring. Because of Dad's illness, I realize that our childhood memories shall never grow old, for the emotion behind them will never lose its comfort to our souls.

Alzheimer's is like a thief in the night, ultimately stealing a person's mind. For the caregiver, however, there are lessons to be learned. If I've learned anything from this experience, it is to enjoy the precious gift of memories that I am able to share with my own daughters.

These gifts can be tucked away in a corner of their middle-aged hearts, to comfort them later, at a time when life might find them becoming a parent to me.

Kathy Gade Whirity
Chicago, Illinois

Those are MY Leaves

We are transplanted Kansans, having spent the best part of our married life raising our family in Lincoln, Nebraska. Even though Lincoln is the second largest city in the state, it has kept many of its small town values. For instance, you can cash a personal check almost anywhere, and if you're standing in line at a restaurant, by the time you reach your table everyone is talking with one another. Neighbors help neighbors. It's just a nice place to be.

Ron and I were married when we were still in high school. The year was 1943, during the Second World War. Upon reaching their eighteenth birthday boys were being removed from their senior class to fill the quotas given their local draft boards. We convinced our folks that getting married was the right thing for us to do. Ron left to serve in the Navy for the next three-and-a-half years. That young marriage, that our families said would never last, has now survived for fifty-eight years! The thing that finally separated us, the thing neither of us could lick, was a progressive disease.

After several years of what was very likely simple Alzheimer's, my husband developed a variation discovered by Fritz Lewy. It is called Lewy Body Dementia. Since these thumb-sized growths have been discovered it is now thought that they develop in the brains of a large percentage of those with Alzheimer's. Lewy Body Dementia progresses more rapidly than Alzheimer's and the symptoms are far more severe. Also the medication often causes serious side effects, making treatment of Lewy a challenge.

During the last year that I was able to keep Ron at home he had become extremely distrustful. He had also reached a point where he had to be constantly on the move. It became such an obsession with him that he seldom ever rested.

Our yard was never so well cared for as it was that summer. He mowed the yard every day and come fall it became a joke in the neighborhood that each time a leaf fell, Ron was out there picking it up. Each Thursday evening everyone on our block sets yard waste out on the curb for Friday morning pick up.

We have two mature maple trees in our backyard. Ron had collected nine large bags of leaves. He lined them up at the curb well before dusk. Each time a car went past or a neighborhood child shouted he would rush to our picture window to be sure no one was stealing his leaves. After dark he went out to count the bags so he could be sure they were all there.

Finally, I could stand it no longer. I said, "Ron, why do we care if someone steals our leaves? They are trash and we want to get rid of them."

Surprised, he exclaimed, "Marian, I can't believe you! Those are *my* leaves and I have the right to give them to whomever I want to give them to, and I want to give them to the garbage man."

Having said that, he carried each bag back to our patio and got up at four the next morning to set them out again.

Marian Summers
Lincoln, Nebraska

Ladies Out For a Ride

Two elderly women were taking an afternoon drive in a luxury car. Both could barely see over the dashboard. As they were cruising along, they came to an intersection. The stoplight was red, but they just went through.

The woman in the passenger seat thought, I must be losing it—I could have sworn we just went through a red light. After a few more minutes they came to another intersection. The light was red, and again they went right through.

This time the passenger was almost certain that the light had been red, but she was also concerned that she might be seeing things. She was getting nervous and decided to pay very close attention.

At the next intersection, sure enough, the light was definitely red and again they went through. She turned to the other woman and said, "Mildred! Did you know we just drove through three red lights in a row? You could have killed us."

Mildred turned to her and said, "Oh, $#!%! Am I driving?"

Anonymous

SECTION THREE

STRANGERS NO MORE

Sometimes life gets so hectic we feel like we are suffering from dementia! How frustrating it is to forget ... to realize that something must be wrong because you cannot remember. How scary it is to not know anyone and want to go home. Where is home? Every place you look is strange and unfamiliar. How did some of your things get here? Where are the rest of your things? And the people, they seem nice, treat you kindly, and even call you by name. *But, who are these people?* This is the reality for our loved ones every day.

Imagine what their lives are like. Imagine what happens when life is so stressful that, as a caregiver, you start forgetting. *Where did I park my car? Oh no, I missed my doctor's appointment! Whom was I supposed to call? Gee, I wish I could remember her name.*

This is why it is important for caregivers to take time off—an afternoon or even a weekend—for respite. This should truly be your FUN time, when you get reenergized. Who knows, your FUN time might also have a positive impact.

What follows are a mix of stories and poems from both perspectives—the person with Alzheimer's (or fast-approaching) and the caregiver's—showing us that there are *strangers no more.*

As caregivers, the more we understand our loved ones' experiences, the less we will feel the stress of uncertainty. And when we take care of ourselves we will have more energy to comfort and care for our loved ones.

The Marriage Proposal

Two active seniors lived in a mobile home park. He was a widower and she was a widow. They had known each other for several years.

One evening, at a community supper in the big activity center, they were seated at a table across from each other. As the meal went on, he made a few admiring glances at her and finally gathered up his courage to ask, "Will you marry me?"

After about six seconds of careful consideration, she answered, "Yes. Yes, I will."

The meal ended and with a few more pleasant exchanges, they went to their respective places.

The next morning he was troubled. "Did she say yes or did she say no?" He couldn't remember. Try as he would, he could not recall. Not even a faint memory.

With trepidation, he went to the telephone and called her. First, he explained that he didn't remember as well as he used to. Then he reviewed the lovely evening past. As he gained a little more courage, he then inquired, "When I asked if you would marry me, did you say yes or did you say no?"

He was delighted to hear her say, "Why, I said, 'Yes. Yes, I will' and I meant it with all my heart." Then she continued, "And I am so glad that you called, because I couldn't remember who had asked me."

Anonymous

A Young Husband

Each night I used to sit outside on the front porch with my friend Marge and her mom, Dorothy. Dorothy was seventy and in the early stages of Alzheimer's. She seemed to enjoy the fresh air and being able to watch the neighborhood kids and adults as they ran or walked by. She had always been a quiet and kind person, who smiled at anyone who came near.

As many people with Alzheimer's do, she repeated the same statements and questions over and over again.

One night Dorothy repeated the same remark about the twenty-three-year old man who lived across the street.

"That's him," she quietly said. "There goes my husband!"

Instead of giving her the same answer we always did—explaining that he wasn't her husband, I decided to try a new approach. "Dorothy," I said, "he can't be your husband. Why, I'm only forty and he's way too young to be *my* husband."

She gave me a long look and huffed, "I'll say!"

She put me right in my place!

Debbie Fisher
Glen Burnie, Maryland

Senility Prayer

God grant me the senility
to forget the people
I never liked anyway,

The good fortune
to run into the ones I do,

And the eyesight
to tell the difference.

Anonymous

That's MY Car!

A petite, elderly lady with finely coiffed white hair finished her shopping. Upon returning to her car, she saw four males getting into her vehicle. She dropped her shopping bags, drew a handgun, and screamed at the top of her voice, "I have a gun, and I will use it! Get out of the car!"

The four men did not wait for a second invitation. They got out and ran like mad. The lady, somewhat shaken, proceeded to load her shopping bags into the back of the car and got into the driver's seat. Still jittery, she struggled to fit her key into the ignition. She tried and tried—and then it dawned on her why.

Noticing an oversized pair of athletic shoes on the passenger-side floor and a crumbled up jacket on the seat, she started looking around the parking lot. Her car was parked four spaces away.

She loaded the bags into her car and then drove to the police station.

The sergeant to whom she apologetically told the story nearly fell over laughing. He pointed to the end of the counter, where four pale men, one in stocking feet and another in a T-shirt, were reporting a car jacking by a mad, elderly woman described as white, less than five feet tall, glasses, curly white hair, and carrying a large handgun.

No charges were filed.

Anonymous
Edited version

(Editor's Note: Another version of this story aired on the CBS television series "Judging Amy.")

Thank you, GOFers

On our recent trip to the Gathering of Friends (GOF) in Nashville, we were lovingly welcomed and repeatedly thanked for bringing our son Kevin to town. You see, Kevin is the Webmaster of TheRibbon.com, a website dedicated to providing support for caregivers who have loved ones suffering from Alzheimer's and dementia. For the last three years Kev has combined his computer savvy with the many talents of a dedicated group of online friends to make the site a reality. These people from across the country were meeting face-to-face for the first time.

The weekend was everything we could have hoped for, and then some. These ladies are so special, caring, funny, and real. We never felt so at home on a trip. All weekend the thank-yous kept coming, to us and to Kev, for all the work he had done. Even though we couldn't agree more that Kev had done a great job with his part of The Ribbon, we began to realize that something was amiss here.

Have any of you wonderful people ever stopped to think about what *you* have done for Kevin?

At a time when Kevin's abilities were frequently hampered by his age (he began working on TheRibbon.com site when he was only fourteen), Karen and Jamie, co-founders of *The Ribbon* newsletter trusted him to showcase the valuable work they were already doing. They welcomed his ideas, and treated him with kindness and respect. They taught him that good people working together can make a difference in others' lives. Thank you for the huge leap of faith you took!

Linda, founder of The Gathering Place site on TheRibbon.com, says, "I hate kids. Just hate them!" Yet,

Linda, we witnessed your respect and kindness while working with Kevin. You are a unique personality (that's a compliment, really!) strong, yet compassionate. And, Kev has learned that people are not always as they first appear!

Then there are the new friends we met in Nashville. For example, Loraine, who walked all twenty-seven laps in the Alzheimer's walk we attended, despite her poor health. She did this because she had made a promise. (We're not sure if it was to herself or someone else.) We will never forget how upset she was when friends talked her into sitting down for even a few minutes, and her determination to get back up and continue. Nor will we forget her Ribbon friends, who made sure she didn't walk one step alone. Thank you for a lesson in courage.

Finally, there are all the ladies we met, who care daily for their loved ones. We are amazed at the tireless dedication you show, your willingness to give up part, or most of your lives, to care for someone else. Seeing you is a touching reminder of watching our mom take care of Dad at home for sixteen years after he had a massive stroke. We did what we could to help her, but never realized how hard it must have been and how many sacrifices she made. Thank you for helping us to see so clearly.

So, thank you. Y'all (Oops, there's that Nashville talk kicking in!) have taught Kevin lessons he will never learn from a book. This is *real* life, and he's learned that the things that matter most come from the heart. We, his parents, thank each of you more than you will ever know.

Debbie and Danny Fisher
Glen Burnie, Maryland

Dreams Do Come True

It took me a year to digest the wonderful events of the 2001 Gathering Of Friends (GOF)—a biannual meeting of care-givers from across the country. There were so many wonderful things in those three brief days of laughter, love, support, and new friendships, that to pinpoint a defining moment is difficult. In fact, when I first sat down to put pen to paper, the original story was five pages long.

Before GOF '01, I tried very hard to convince Mary, a friend who is more like a sister to me, that she needed to attend this event. I told her it would be the break she needed following her mother's death as it would help her deal with the grief. I spent many nights on the phone and on the Internet trying to persuade her. Mary was unwavering in her belief that no one wanted to be around her or to hear about *Ma*, whom she had cared for in her home for five years. I emphasized that there was a place and a purpose for her in Nashville; but Mary insisted she was not coming. She even went so far as to tell me to quit asking, I was making her mad!

The night before the trip, I was on the phone with Mary, begging and pleading in a last ditch effort—offering my last *Hail Mary* prayer. *Nope, no dice*, she would hear none of it! At the end of our conversation, I told Mary, "Well, I'm not giving up hope, dreams do come true!"

After a long day of flying and anticipation, the plane finally touched down at the Nashville airport. As I stepped onto the escalator, heading down to baggage claim, I saw Jamie, our hostess for the weekend. She was standing there with a huge grin. Hugging her, I asked hopefully, "Did she (Mary) come?" The answer to my question was lost in all the excitement of introductions, hugs, confusion, and luggage to claim.

It seemed my hopes and dreams were for naught. I just knew Mary would be here; I felt it. Though it appeared I was wrong. I was crushed, heartbroken. I had a brief talk with myself, "Okay, get a grip here. It will be a fun weekend, just make up your mind to enjoy it."

We made our way to the car rental counter. There were two customers ahead of us, so everyone was jabbering away getting to know each other better. Laughing and joking, the respite weekend was off to a grand start. Jamie and I were putting together some last-minute plans for the weekend, when I heard a woman's voice shriek that she had to get a car *now*! I spun around to see what the problem was—and it was Mary! A huge red bow was tied around her neck and she was giggling like a child. I do not recall what was said. All I know is we were wiping tears of joy from our eyes. As our tears turned into giggles and snickers, one by one the gang informed me they had been in on the surprise all along.

I had no clue. I had been strung along like this for *months*! I didn't care! I knew then that the weekend would be everything it was intended to be, and more.

A full agenda of activities included the primary event— the Alzheimer's Memory Walk (the funds our team raised benefitted the Central Nashville Chapter). Participating in the walk was one of the more healing moments for Mary and for most of us.

Our group attracted attention with our matching shirts that were captioned with *Jane's Angels—Helping to Pay it*

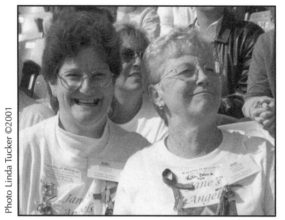

Photo Linda Tucker ©2001

Jamie Aguilar and Karen Bradley, co-founders of TheRibbon.com

Forward. (Jane Levy, AlzJane198 to those who knew her on the Internet for her participation in Alzheimer's chat rooms, was an inspiration. Her memory continues to inspire those who care for loved ones with Alzheimer's. Sadly, Jane passed away in February 1999. We named the team in her honor.) The back of our shirts advertised TheRibbon.com and The Gathering Place (www.TheRibbon.com—Alzheimer's newsletter website and www.TheRibbon.com/GatherPlace —an Alzheimer's chat room for caregiver support). Inquisitive walkers asked us questions before the walk began and we happily answered and explained about the Internet caregiver support opportunities.

Following the opening ceremonies at Greer Stadium, home of the Nashville Sound Baseball team, the walking teams were called out to the field. The announcer asked for *Jane's Angels* to lead the honorary lap. The announcer explained to the 600-plus walkers that we had come from across the country for this weekend of respite and that we had met on the Internet. Many of us were meeting in person for the first time. *What an honor for our group of eighteen folks. Our hearts swelled with pride and, of course, there were more tears!*

The rest of the weekend was a whirlwind of activity. As we formed new friendships, I noticed Mary blooming like a flower. The heavy burden that weighed in her heart lightened with each passing minute. She was milling about, answering people's questions about *Jane's Angels*, and making sure to take time with each of us before we started the walk. (She gave us bottles of bubbles so that we could blow bubbles for a pre-walk icebreaker.) This weekend was Mary's time to heal—to rediscover that she *did* matter and what she said was important.

In fact, I witnessed our entire group blossom over the weekend—from the first meeting at the airport, the Meet-and-Greet evening at Jamie's, the walk, the barbeque, the Opryland Hotel, finding Art (an innocent bystander who became my dream cowboy for all too brief of a time), and to the last evening of goofing off at the hotel.

On our last morning at the hotel, we took a few minutes to reflect on the wonderful events held during the weekend and we cried more tears. The weekend gave us a stronger sense of our huge accomplishment: caring for our loved ones. The GOF gave us the confidence to feel that, as caregivers, we are truly an amazing bunch, as we give unconditionally of ourselves.

Monday was departure day and our hearts were filled with sadness. After returning to the airport and getting organized, we choked down a bite of lunch. As much as I

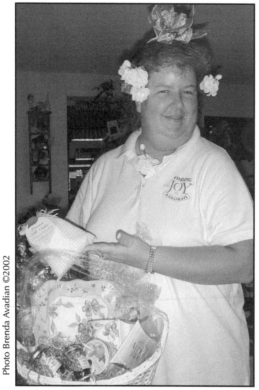

Photo Brenda Avadian ©2002

Linda Tucker enjoys a gift basket filled with FUN. Linda is a long-distance caregiver and founder of The Gathering Place: http://www.theribbon.com/gatherplace/

tried to keep it light and happy, the weak one here—I just couldn't seem to turn off the tears. We tried to put off the inevitable, but the time had come for us to leave. I caught up with Mary and held her hand as we walked to the security checkpoint. We hugged and tearfully said goodbye to our friends who were staying in Nashville.

Mary was the first to leave. Her flight was announced and my tears started flowing again. We hugged and then she pulled out a package wrapped in purple tissue paper and stuffed it into my bag. She grabbed me for one last hug and told me, "Open that *later*. And remember, dreams do come true!" With that, she swirled away and was gone.

As the rest of our group made its way back up the concourse to the next departure gate, I looked at the gals and asked if I could open the box. With their permission, I gently peeled off the purple tissue paper and lifted the lid. Inside the box was a beautiful dream catcher.

That weekend I learned: In spite of all odds—don't give up! Even when the deck seems stacked against you; don't quit dreaming, you might never experience the *unforgettable* joys that could pass you by.

Most of all I learned: Dreams do come true!

Linda Tucker
Northern California

A Lady's Bequest

What do you see, nurses, what do you see?
What are you thinking when you're looking at me?
A crabby old woman, not very wise,
Uncertain of habit, with faraway eyes?
Who dribbles her food and makes no reply
When you say in a loud voice, "I do wish you'd try!"
Who seems not to notice the things that you do,
And forever is losing a stocking or shoe.
Who, resisting or not, lets you do as you will,
With bathing and feeding, the long day to fill.
Is that what you're thinking? Is that what you see?
Then open your eyes, nurse; you're not looking at me.
I'll tell you who I am as I sit here so still,
As I do your bidding, as I eat at your will.
I'm a small child of ten . . . with a father and mother,
Brothers and sisters, who love one another.
A young girl of sixteen, with wings on her feet,
Dreaming that soon now a lover she'll meet.
A bride soon at twenty—my heart gives a leap,
Remembering the vows that I promised to keep.
At twenty-five now, I have young of my own,
Who need me to guide and a secure, happy home.
A woman of thirty, my young now grown fast,
Bound to each other with ties that should last.
At forty, my young sons are grown and have gone,
But my man's beside me to see I don't mourn.
At fifty, once more babies play around my knee,
Again we know children, my loved one and me.
Dark days are upon me, my husband is dead;

I look at the future, I shudder with dread.
For my young are rearing young of their own,
And I think of the years and the love that I've known.
I'm now an old woman . . . and nature is cruel;

'Tis jest to make old age look like a fool.
The body, it crumbles, grace and vigor depart.
There is now a stone where I once had a heart.
But inside this old carcass a young girl still dwells,
And now and again my battered heart swells.
I remember the joys. I remember the pain.
And I'm loving and living life over again.
I think of the years . . . all too few, gone too fast,
And accept the stark fact that nothing can last.

So open your eyes, nurses, open and see,
not a crabby old woman; look closer . . . see ME!!

(Editor's Note: This poem was written by an elderly woman who died in the geriatric ward of a small hospital in Dundee, Scotland. After her death, the nurses found the poem when they were going through her meager possessions. The quality and content of the poem impressed them so much that copies were made and distributed to every nurse in the hospital—and beyond. The poem and this explanation eventually circled the Internet, where we found it.)

The Neighbor's Bathroom?

The hospital room was quiet and dim. The only sound was Donald's labored breathing. At some point in the long hours of waiting, someone appeared in the doorway. It was the doctor announcing to me that my husband had Alzheimer's disease.

Okay. So the illness had a name, finally. Big deal. But what does it mean? The doctor's reply blew me away.

"It's a fatal disease," I heard. "No known cause and no known cure."

"What am I to do?"

"Just take him home and wait for him to die."

Suddenly I felt crazed, insane, dumbheaded, numb, enraged, hysterical—all at once! What am I supposed to do? Where do I go for help? Who can offer help and advice? Why has this happened to *my* Donald?

Until this moment I had always thought depression was simply a deep and abiding sadness. And it is. But the depression is overwhelming in its scope. Sapping energy, intelligence, clear thinking . . . and on top of the horror of the doctor's statement, I now must assume the responsibilities and burdens that had always been Donald's. He could no longer drive and I could not leave him alone. I had to do everything with and for him: get the car serviced, buy groceries, write the checks, pay the bills, dial the telephone, turn the TV on or off, etc. Donald had always kept my kitchen knives sharpened. He no longer knew how to do a job he had done for sixty years. I had to take over the myriad little things I had never expected to do.

I had a new "kid" on my hands. It was time for me to

figure out a way to contend with this dreadful Alzheimer's disease.

Although I grew depressed watching Donald deteriorate, I needed to find a way to function. Once upon a time, I had been told that we should find something humorous in every intolerable situation. Humor helps me to acknowledge and endure what is otherwise unendurable.

A line from a poem by Marion Doyle that I heard years ago came to mind:

> *Tears will quench the first white flame of grief*
> *When laughter is a thing beyond belief.*
> *But strangest of all strange things that are . . .*
> *Laughter is balsam for the scar.*

Taking this as my shibboleth, I began to see the humor in some of the more ridiculous events in our lives.

❧ ❧

Donald shuffled into the kitchen, where I was quite busy. He announced, in a childlike way, that he wanted to go to the bathroom . . . almost asking for permission.

"Okay," I said. "Go to the bathroom."

"I don't know where it is," he replied.

"Just down the hall . . ."

Donald had been gone for a while when I noticed that our apartment door was open. He had crossed the hallway to a nearby apartment and they would not let him use their bathroom. Always a very neat, clean, and modest person, Donald was greatly embarrassed as his need became more imperative. Fortunately, our other neighbor heard the ruckus in the hallway and was kind and understanding. He brought Donald home. I took Donald to our *own* bathroom, in our *own* apartment.

With great delight he exclaimed, "Isn't this wonderful? We have a bathroom of our *own*! And it is so clean. And it is right here in our own place!"

He was ecstatic! I laughed. Our neighbor laughed. Donald laughed. For a brief moment there was laughter in our lives.

Evelyn Daniel
Lancaster, California

Frannie Bell

She was little,
she was,
with red-brown hair,
and girlish freckles yet,
small gold-rimmed glasses;
mostly smiling,
her face showed no pain.
She read with her
book upside down
on her breast. She
read all day, every day,
in her hospital room.

Which failed first?
Her mind or her heart?
I never can recall. Her
papers said, "Alzheimer's."
Secondary diagnosis:
heart failure.

She came and went
again and again,
in and out of the ER
doors, given Life
to live though she
possessed no memory.

Yet, one day
she rose, leaving
her book on her

bed sheets, and she
crossed the room
alone and straight.
She never wobbled.

Frannie Bell
put her arms
around a sobbing
woman and said
quite clearly:
"There, there, Dear.
Don't cry. Tears
won't change a thing."

Then Frannie turned.
She went back to her bed.
She picked up her book.
She read upside down,
unknowing, staring
out the window
between the pages.

f. Hannah
Granada Hills, California

Did You Ever Dream ...

that to Nashville
you would go?
For some, not only once,
but two times or so?

that you would meet
that special screen name at long last,
whose face now will remain
in your mind ever so fast?

that the hugs seen on the screen,
which you longed to feel
are now felt live,
so wonderfully real?

that in helping to *pay it forward*,
Jane's Angels would be asked
to lead the Honorary Lap?
And then, as a team,
complete the Alzheimer's Memory Walk
hand-in-hand with nary a gap?

that an evening of remembering our
friends and loved ones here and past
was mixed with daring
to hope for a cure to come at long last?

that releasing balloons—
rising so high in the sky
would bring precious memories of
dear Jane to our mind's eye?

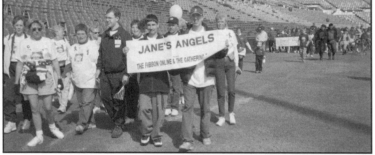

Photo Linda Tucker ©2001

Jane's Angels start the Memory Walk in Nashville, Tennessee

that during an excursion to the Opryland Hotel
you would find a dream of a cowboy named Art,
who laughed and smiled—
wasn't he just really swell?

that a night of
laughter and cheer
could be mixed with
so many healing tears?

that now with the dreaded
day of departure here,
you dare feel JOY in your heart as you know your
new friends will be there to help ease those daily fears?

that you had dared to dream your soul friend/adopted
twin
would surprise you by coming on this trip
and now sadly walking to her gate, holding her hand,
not wanting to let go of her grip?

that even though this weekend of fun and
tears had to come to an end,
there is no longer a need to dare to
dream or even to pretend?

The proof is now written
to last for all time.
You see, *dreams do come true*
thanks to seventeen friends
and an adopted twin of mine.

*Remembering The Second Biannual Gathering of Friends
Sponsored by TheRibbon.com and The Gathering Place
October 5-8, 2001-Nashville, Tennessee*

Linda Tucker
Northern California

Section Four

TRIBUTES

*H*ow many of us can honestly say that our lives have not been altered in some way by caring for our loved ones? The caregiver whose life has not dramatically changed is rare. Hopefully among the tears there are joyful moments we recall that help us stay strong enough to get through each day. Some of these moments remain and we find ourselves remembering them weeks, months, and even years later.

While I was compiling information for the first volume of *Finding the JOY in Alzheimer's: Caregivers Share the Joyful Times,* caregivers expressed their appreciation for being included. They felt their stories would help other caregivers and that being in print was one way of paying tribute to their families and friends.

Although most of the stories, poems, and photos in this volume could appropriately be included in this part of the book, I had to limit the number of entries in this largest section. What follows are submissions from husbands about their wives, daughters about their mothers, wives writing about their husbands, a ten-year old writing about Grandpa, and friends paying tribute to friends.

To My Wife

While on vacation with our daughter's family during the summer of 1996, I realized that Gail, my wife of over forty years, might have Alzheimer's.

The clue seemed inconsequential. We were planning to drive home and wanted to visit relatives along the way. Gail always carried a small black phone book in her purse. She pulled it out and read a phone number to me. It only had six digits and after several minutes of conversation, she could not understand that we needed seven digits. Gail already had what I thought were normal lapses in memory associated with aging. But since her mother had Alzheimer's (it was confirmed by an autopsy) and her grandmother, five aunts and uncles, and one cousin, had the same symptoms; my mind wouldn't let me be optimistic.

When we returned home, Gail went through a complete battery of tests, all of which indicated early-onset Alzheimer's. Then we began to deal with the diagnosis one-day-at a time.

❧ ❧

Forty years ago, Gail and I met and married in Dallas, Texas. After our first date we knew we were in love. We adored each other; we were always sensitive to each other's needs and remained each other's best friend. We never wanted to be away from each other.

Gail's father deserted the family when Gail was ten years old. Although she helped her mother raise two younger siblings, Gail was able to create another life with high school friends who provided her with strong emotional support through the years.

Gail did not attend college because the family struggled financially. For the first several years we were married, she worked in various positions with Exxon Mobil. After our first child was born, she became a full-time, loving, nurturing, and caring mother. Gail stayed home until both of our children went off to college.

From the time we were married and until she became ill, Gail was devoted to the church, particularly to the children's Sunday school program. She started out as a Sunday school teacher and later became head of the entire children's program at a church that has several thousand members. Eventually Gail was a paid staff member at the church.

Later she worked for ten years as a teacher's aide in the pre-school program for ages three and four. She loved the children as if they were her own.

Gail was also active in the Disciples Study Fellowship, having studied in a yearlong program before she and a close friend started a program at our church, which is still in operation today. Outside of family-related activities and working with children, this was the most satisfying accomplishment of Gail's life.

Before Alzheimer's started taking its toll, Gail always seemed to say what was appropriate in every situation. She was an excellent public speaker and she could introduce twenty to thirty people without missing a name. She was a lovely, warm, and caring wife, mother, and friend—a remarkable person.

🌿 🌿

Of all the experiences we have had since Gail was diagnosed, the following one touches my heart and soul more than any other.

Gail was at the stage where she often didn't know who I was. One morning I had just finished helping her take a shower. I was holding her as she got out of the shower and was softly drying her, including all the places that previously were sensual. At only sixty-four Gail still had a cute body.

All of a sudden, she stood straight up, completely nude, and looked up into my eyes. Parts of her still not-yet-dried body glistened. She said feelingly, caringly, and with conviction, "You sure are a nice man." Then she paused for a few seconds, as if thinking. Then said very lovingly and somewhat apologetically, "But I love my husband."

For an instant tears welled up, but I knew I didn't want to cry in front of her and I was also aware of *validation therapy*, which essentially says to validate what the person is saying. I simply said, "That's okay," and nothing more was said. Then I realized this was one of those happy-sad-happy-sad moments that you never forget and it helped me appreciate who she was, a kind and loving wife whom I have been blessed with for almost fifty years. Later, I did cry (as I am doing now); but after a while I will laugh and relive that precious moment.

Gail is now in the advanced stage of Alzheimer's and is in a nursing facility in Austin, Texas. The Alzheimer's Association here is staffed with angels. They adopted us two years ago when we moved from our home and friends of thirty years in Houston to be closer to our son. Without their kindness, understanding, and constant support, we would not have survived.

Since Gail has been in the nursing facility, I have more time to devote to church and its missionary outreach. Additionally I am helping other families deal with Alzheimer's. First, I get them in touch with the Alzheimer's

Association. If they hesitate, I don't pressure them, but I don't give up either. I also visit them during the week and even call during the day.

Despite the feelings of joy at being able to help others through these times of uncertainty, there are moments when the memories of my own most challenging times come flooding back and almost overwhelm me. But, I couldn't live with myself if I didn't help others because I have been there and I know I can make a difference.

Less stressful is assisting the Alzheimer's Association in any way I can. I have been on a panel discussion on Alzheimer's that they sponsored. Also, I have lobbied members of the Texas legislature, with the Association's staff, and testified before the Texas Department of Human Services on bills that would affect Alzheimer's families—all coordinated by the Association's government relations official.

Whatever else I may do, however, is *a drop in the bucket* compared to the support our family has received from the Austin chapter.

Jerry L. Gibson
Austin, Texas

My Mother's Touch

She cradled me and marveled at me

She sang to me, held my hand and comforted me

She cleaned up my spills and forgave me for everything

She made my Christmas stocking

She smocked my dresses and curled my straight hair

She led my Brownie Troop and taught my Sunday
school classes

She wiped my tears and bandaged my wounds

She offered to help me pack when I threatened to run
away from home

She listened to my heartaches and joys and calmed my
fears

She watched me dance and drove me to piano lessons

She promised me my little brother would stop picking
on me someday

She protected me and she let me run

She always kissed me good-night and hugged me a lot

She encouraged and nurtured me, prayed for me and
showed me a way

She sat close to me, stood by me and understood me

She worried about me every day of her life

But most of all, she taught me about love.

She drew me into God's love, to sit in God's lap, and be
wrapped in the love of the Mother God.

And she did this with so many children—touching their
lives with her gentle squeeze, her infectious loving smile,

and her joyful heart that sparkled in her pretty blue eyes.

How many years of Sunday school classes, School for Little People and neighborhood children? Only God will be able to count how many when God sees Mom's fingerprints of love on each of their hearts.

What has lived and loved in her does not diminish, but lives on in each of us. Her light, which never hid under a bushel, shines in my children, in my brother and his children, in many others, and me.

She is an angel passing through this world, reminding us that children need all our love and care, attention, and protection.

Her spirit of kindness and generosity embraced us every day.

Sallie Gibson Holmes
Silver Spring, Maryland

(Jerry Gibson writes: Our daughter, Sallie, wrote a loving tribute to her mother in honor of Gail's 67th birthday on July 27, 2001. Gail was not able to understand it, but for our family it is a beautiful reflection of who she was, and still is, to us.)

Jerry's Dream

In 1995, my husband was in the process of getting his pilot's license. He and two other partners owned a small airplane. To fly an airplane was one of his lifelong dreams. He worked hard at it and was very close to getting his license. Then, he was diagnosed with Early Onset Alzheimer's Disease (EOAD) and it was strongly suggested that he discontinue his effort.

It wasn't an easy task to persuade him to give up his flying lessons. Since he was early into the disease, I think he finally realized on his own that he couldn't continue. His partnership was sold and I sadly believed this would be the end of his dream.

But, he continued having his dream, only on a smaller scale. Years earlier one of his hobbies was constructing and flying remote-control airplanes. Each of these planes had patiently been sanded, painted, and put together piece-by-piece. At this time, he didn't have any of the planes, which he had devoted so much of his spare time to. So, he happily started over.

We decided to buy one that was ready to fly because I was fairly sure that he would find it difficult to construct one as he had before. We bought the plane and it was ready to go—but he wasn't. It took him months to get up enough nerve to take it out and fly. He finally did, and it crashed.

I have to say that was probably the end of any hands-on type of flying. The broken, crashed plane is still hanging in his workshop and occasionally he will point it out to me, either with a smile from a happy memory or sadness from the final, unhappy one.

His dream continues. He loves anything that flies. Sometimes it can be quite comical to watch him. It doesn't matter what time of day or night, with the excitement of a small child, he can spot any flying object. Our family and friends have become quite used to the fact that if he spots something in flight, he must point it out to us. And, we must react as if we are as excited as he is. Of course, the grandchildren enjoy seeing planes fly as much as he does—no pretending is necessary on their part.

I often wonder what onlookers think, especially when there are no children with us. In my opinion, it must look funny.

It does not matter; Jerry has his dream tucked away, somewhere in his mind. He still seems to enjoy these memories and he has given us a pleasant memory to tuck in our minds. This memory brings us joy and makes us laugh each time we look up into the day or night sky and see an airplane flying. We will think of Jerry, a devoted husband, father and friend, who held on to his dream as long as he could.

❋   ❋

Postscript: Since I wrote this story, about a year ago, Jerry had to be placed in a nursing home. I believe he may have lost his dream of flying. Today, however, we hold a very precious memory. All of us, especially the grandchildren, laugh and giggle each time we notice one of Jerry's dreams flying overhead. Among the many, many, wonderful memories we have of Jerry, his dream of flying is one of our favorites.

Sharon DeMoe
Beggs, Oklahoma

A Shining Knight

My husband, Bruce, was diagnosed with Alzheimer's in October 1999. One month later, he had a severe stroke. In spite of his inability to function, Bruce's doctor would not admit him to the hospital. Whether this was due to Bruce having Alzheimer's, I don't know. I cared for Bruce at home with the help of home-health care and many wonderful neighbors.

I thought I was giving him excellent care. I was not aware that lying on his back so much and sitting up so little would cause pneumonia. Bruce was admitted to the hospital in February. I knew I was unable to care for him on his release, so I placed him in a nursing home.

When Bruce was admitted into the nursing home he weighed eighty-four pounds. He could not talk or walk and he didn't respond much in any way. The staff immediately began to work vigorously with him. In six months they had Bruce functional—to the point of being a problem! They never knew one minute to the next where he would be or what he would be doing.

In the wing where Bruce lived were two sisters. Isabel was ninety-one and Madeline was a few years older. Madeline was very quiet and rarely came out of her room except to eat. Isabel was the opposite. Some days I would see her rolling up and down the halls with a sweet smile on her face and a pleasant greeting for everyone. Other days she would be giving the world a tongue lashing at the top of her lungs.

One morning, the staff could hardly wait for me to come visit. Mind you, my husband is a southern gentleman and very macho. These two sisters almost always had their own private table in the nursing home dining room as long as there were not too many patients. This one particular day, a new patient came in and was placed at their table. Well, Isabel was not going to stand for that. She proceeded to berate the newcomer and soon had her crying.

Upon seeing a woman in tears my husband was on his white charger and dashed to the rescue. He was only one hundred pounds and could barely walk. Isabel was a large woman, perhaps close to one hundred seventy-five pounds. He got up from his chair, tottered over, grabbed hold of Isabel's wheelchair, and proceeded to roll her back to her room. The staff heard him tell Isabel that she could stay in her room until she behaved herself.

The entire nursing home was delighted. All those who had not witnessed the episode told me they wished so much they could have seen it too. I asked if Isabel had stayed in her room. Much to my surprise, they said she did.

Lorraine H. Tucker
Pharr, Texas

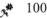

A Secret Communication

A special bond has always existed between my mom, who had Alzheimer's, and my grandson. When Alex was two, they seemed to be at the same point in their lives.

I'd watch, amazed, as Mother and Alex revealed similar capabilities while feeding themselves, communicating, and comprehending. Alex touched my mom's arm with his hand. Mother smiled and patted his head.

Alex sat in the wheelchair with her. Mother jabbered in contentment, while Alex gazed into her eyes.

Mother began to need someone to feed her. Alex was starting to feed himself competently.

Mother continued to grow backward and Alex moved forward.

Alex always told us that Great Grandma DeeDee was talking to him when she made unintelligible (to us) sounds, not words. When she smiled, he insisted it was a smile for him.

Could they communicate? We don't know, but Alex seemed to comfort and calm the older woman, and his world was brightened when she smiled and made sounds.

Whenever we visited my mother, he played contentedly around her room at the nursing home; sometimes with his older sister, sometimes by himself. He seldom declined an invitation to accompany me.

Alex is now almost six years old. During his last visit, Mother, who hardly ever responded to us anymore, was having one of her better days and made sounds. Alex said she was talking with him. He also insisted she was humming to the music playing on the radio in her room.

He has this memory to carry him along since her death a few months ago, for he seems to miss her more than anyone. We discuss Grandma DeeDee and recall our visits with her.

"She talked to me," Alex recalls and smiles, as we put together a memory book of this lady who, unknowingly, has played such an important role in his young life.

Mary Emma Allen
Plymouth, New Hampshire

(Editor's Note: This story appeared in 2theheart.com ezine —electronic magazine)

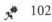

Answer the Coffee Cup?

As near as I can figure, Jim was six to seven years into the disease and was frustrated at not being able to communicate. Also, he was quite often short-tempered.

It was late afternoon. I was in the kitchen starting to prepare dinner and Jim was in his chair in the living room. He had been agitated all day. I had brought him some coffee earlier and was glad that he seemed to have calmed down a little.

The phone rang. As I was starting to wipe the flour off my hands to answer it, I heard Jim say, "Hello." He said it once, twice, and then again, getting louder each time. But the phone kept ringing. Before long, he was angrily shouting, "HELLO!" Meanwhile, the phone continued to ring.

I peered around the corner into the living room and there was Jim, holding the coffee cup to his ear, shouting into thin air, while coffee dripped from his ear, to his lowered chin, and onto his chest.

The whole thing just struck me so funny, that I had to return to the kitchen. Grabbing a towel, I put it over my face and had the best laugh I'd had in a long time.

I know this sounds cruel, but under the constant stress of caregiving, you either laugh or cry and I had already cried enough.

Helen Bennett Jones
Lancaster, California

(Editor's Note: Helen passed away unexpectedly, shortly before her husband's passing. During the time we knew her, she reminded us to laugh. This story is included in her memory.)

103

A Ten-Year-Old Makes a Difference

My Grandpa Dick and a lot of other people have a disease called Alzheimer's. Alzheimer's is a disease that makes you forget how to feed yourself. When I go to visit Grandpa I always ask him, "Have you been a good boy?"

Sometimes he will say, "Yep" and sometimes he will say, "Nope" because he has this terrible disease.

Alzheimer's can be a happy or a sad time. When it is a good and happy time for Grandpa, he will respond to us. When he is sad or upset he might not respond, but he knows that we are right there beside him. I love to visit Grandpa because he is a nice man and I love him very much.

I started thinking about a good way to raise money for this terrible disease. My twin brother, Jeremy, and I came up with the idea of raising funds at a golf course after going to a family reunion. We could make a miniature golf course in our backyard! When we got home we talked to some neighbor kids and they said they would help us with the course. Jeremy, my sister, Jennifer, and I did most of it. Jeremy and I put the course together using bricks and wood scraps from around our house. The bricks helped support the wood so that we could make golf balls bounce off the wood.

We made advertisements and put them up around our neighborhood and the post office. We also asked friends, family, and neighbors. Our step dad asked people at his work, too. A round of golf would be fifty cents.

When people saw the advertisements for the golf course, they came to see what we had put together. When we tried to give people change they would tell us not to give them any. One person even gave us ten dollars! By putting the golf course together we raised fifty dollars for the Alzheimer's Memory Walk. Mom surprised us by calling the newspaper. A lady came and interviewed us and took our picture. The lady who interviewed us told us to look in the newspaper. We were really surprised to see a story about the golf course and our picture in the paper.

Every September my family raises money and then walks in the Alzheimer's Memory Walk. This year we walked, too. There is a four-mile walk, but you can walk as far as you would like. This is the fourth year that we have walked, and this is the fifth year my mom has been on the Alzheimer's Memory Walk committee.

Jason Williams
Oneida, Illinois

As Time Goes By

When my grandmother passed away I felt like I had already been mourning for over a year. Alzheimer's is a cruel disease that robs us of our loved ones, little by little, memory-by-memory. Loretta Everding was a strong German woman, until her eightieth year. What began as moments of confusion would eventually lead up to a nearly total lack of comprehension.

In between we managed to go on living, loving, and even laughing. Grandma wasn't one to feel sorry for herself and she'd get mad at you if you felt sorry for her. She always said, "Remember me with smiles and laughter, or don't remember me at all." It was part of a poem she had photocopied for all of us grandchildren years ago. So in honor of her and at her insistence, I relay a short story of her antics under the influence of Alzheimer's.

⁕ ⁕

Grandma's medications made her sleepy at times and on many occasions she would fall asleep in her armchair while she watched the evening news. Now, truthfully, she had always done this, but usually it was the late night news that she fell asleep watching. But she liked to blame things on her medicine, so this is how the story goes.

As the year passed and the days got shorter, by the time the evening news ended it was dark outside. When Grandma awoke, she would look out the window and see the darkness that had not been there when she began resting her eyes. She assumed it was morning, the light just beginning rather than fading, and that she had slept in her chair all night long. Of course this wasn't true. She had only been asleep for about twenty minutes.

Grandma would jump up and let the dog out, thinking Brittany must be desperate to relieve herself. Then, Grandma would become quite flustered when Brittany just sniffed around, since she'd only just been outside about an hour earlier.

The *morning* would progress with coffee and very dark toast. Again Brittany would be a cause for frustration, by turning her nose up at *breakfast*, since she'd just eaten dinner. Grandma would then get dressed for her art class and be ready to go, waiting to be picked up by a friend who could still drive a car. Then she noticed, while waiting at the window, that it was getting darker not lighter outside. The clock said 8:00. Was it a.m. or p.m.? Picking up the phone Grandma called my aunt and asked her if it was morning or evening. Of course, my aunt told her it was evening, and Grandma had a good laugh at herself, but then had to get ready for bed all over again.

This happened so often that we all wondered what we could possibly do to help. My aunt, being the most affected, decided to purchase a special clock for Grandma. You never had to set it. It had an internal computer or something and it was in tune with the universal clock. It had a big a.m. and p.m. display and also told the day of the week, the date, and the year. We all thought it was wonderful. Well, all of us except for Grandma.

Whenever she fell asleep in her chair, and she thought it was morning when she awoke, she took one look at that clock and her stubborn German blood took over. She KNEW it was morning, yet the clock told her it was evening. She tried again and again to change the settings on that clock, but couldn't do it.

I now have the clock and I smile every time I look at it, recalling how Grandma would call me and tell me how she'd done it again, and then she'd say, "Wasn't life funny?"

Maybe I'll call my aunt and ask her what year it is, just to give her a smile.

Heather Froeschl
Callaway, Virginia

Happy Mother's Day

I have a deep love for my mother, who was diagnosed with Alzheimer's disease in 1998. It seemed to come on suddenly, when she was staying with my brother. That I might be losing my mother was the most painful realization of my life. We decided to move her to Colorado, where I live. I never had a chance to think about it. I knew I had to act.

With time and medication she has settled in and feels comfortable in her new home—the Alzheimer's unit. Mom is like a child, having fun and meeting new people. She likes to dance, and is the life of the party. She has a great sense of humor and a smile that fills the room. My parents divorced when I was a child, so I don't remember her smiling much. In her new home she no longer has worries and is proud to have raised five children, including a set of twins, by herself. She taught us about life and is proud of what we have become.

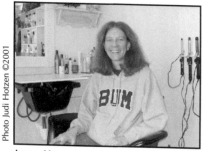

Photo Judi Hotzen ©2001

Lynn Keane sporting a BUM sweatshirt.

I visit and share pictures with her often. Recently I gave her a picture of me wearing a comfortable sweatshirt with a "BUM" logo.

Rather than framing it behind glass, which can be dangerous for the residents, I taped it on the wall. During a later visit I noticed that part of the word "BUM" was missing from the picture. I asked, "Mom, why did you scratch at the picture like that?"

"You're not a bum. You are the best daughter I have," she replied.

My eyes filled with tears. On my next visit I brought new pictures and covered the hole with a different picture. She just smiled, content once again.

Lynn S. Keane
Colorado Springs, Colorado

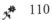

Father's Day

My eighty-two-year-old grandmother had Alzheimer's. Most often she would refer to my Mama as He. I had gone over to Mama's house to help out with Grandmother. While helping Grandmother, Mama and I were discussing Father's Day.

Grandmother, who was hard-of-hearing without her hearing aides, was feeling left out of the conversation. She asked me in a bawdy-broad voice, "Are you going to buy her a Father's Day gift?"

What? A lucid moment? Grandmother was back to being that bawdy-broad we knew her to be while growing up? Mama was actually back to being a she?

I thought for a moment and told Grandmother, "You know what, I should. My mom has been both father and mother to all of us kids for most of our lives."

I don't remember exactly how old I was when my parents divorced, but I do know that my father was not around for most of my life.

Mom wasn't perfect, but she managed to keep a roof over our heads one way or another and some kind of food in our mouths. She worked two or three jobs to support us, so she wasn't able to be home much. On her days off she would take the bunch of us riding around or fishing on Old Hickory Lake.

On Father's Day, I pondered my friend Jan's e-mail signature block— "The Heart Always Remembers" and then followed my mother's example.

I spent time with her and Grandmother. I gave them the

best gift I possibly could so their hearts would remember. I thanked my mother for doing her best for all of us six kids.

Jamie Aguilar
Nashville, Tennessee

(Editor's Note: This story has been edited since it first appeared in TheRibbon.com)

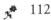

My Love, Forever

Our journey began six years ago when my wife was diagnosed with this horrible disease. Our lives changed dramatically from that moment on. She was fifty-nine and I was fifty-six. We had been married for thirty-five years—a time of happiness and loving each other very much.

We were, as they say, joined at the hip. We have three lovely girls who are having a difficult time dealing with what has happened to their mom.

My life as a husband seemed to come to an end, or at least as a marriage should be. My loving wife, Loretto, went downhill after the initial diagnosis. My health has not been that good either. With the added stress I suffered a heart attack three years ago, and then had bypass surgery. It didn't end there.

Shortly after my surgery, I was hit head-on by a drunk driver resulting in a broken collarbone, dislocated shoulder, collapsed lung, and multiple bruises. The car was totaled.

The effects of the accident, together with the bypass surgery, made it very difficult for me to care for my wife at home. My doctor strongly advised that I place her in a home where she could receive the care I could not provide. I did this over a year ago.

Having never lived alone until that time, adjusting to living at home without a spouse became even worse. Life was very lonely for me.

However, Loretto has settled into the home very well and has made many friends. She has more or less taken ownership of her floor. I have been told she takes the new residents under her wing—comforting and assuring them that everything will be okay. When I visit her she says to whomever she is sitting with, "Here is my honey." Her friends have now become my friends and their faces light up when I walk into the home. Not only does my wife enjoy my daily visits; so do they. When I leave I give my wife a kiss. Other residents ask, "Do I get one of those, too?" I accommodate with a kiss on each of their foreheads.

On the advice of a very dear friend, I have placed a daily diary in Loretto's room. I write happy things in it that we enjoy now. From time-to-time I read the entries to my wife.

A year ago we had our fortieth wedding anniversary and a family gathering at a lodge. At the urging of the same dear friend, we made an event of the occasion. I was in my best suit, with a new tie and a flower in my lapel. My bride looked beautiful. She had her hair done and was adorned in her best dress, with a corsage I had given her earlier in the day. Loretto enjoyed my speech; I do believe she even remembered some of the stories.

The week prior to our anniversary, I had placed our wedding album in her room. Each day I visited, we looked at the album. I told her about the crazy things that had happened on our wedding day. The nurses who visited her room also looked at the album; it helped her remember it was a very special day.

During my more recent visits to the home, Loretto has me lay down on her bed with her. I hold her and tell her things from the past. She tells me she likes this more than anything else she does during the day.

The nurses and staff love Loretto. They say she gives them a reason to smile each day. The truth be told, she brings a smile to my face also. When I visit, she can never be found in her room, she is visiting with other residents, bringing laughter and meaning to their day.

On October 12, 2002, our oldest daughter was married. Loretto and I had a wonderful day with friends and relatives. One of my sons-in-law captured the entire day on video. It was nicely done, so I asked Monica, the recreational administrator, if I could show it to some of the residents. She thought it was a great idea.

I created invitations for twenty of the residents. The home served popcorn and punch. The nurses dressed up Loretto for the day, which made her feel very special. I announced at the beginning that my wife and I wanted to share the video with our new family at the home. Everyone had a very good time. The video was rather long; however, it held their attention to the end. Today, the residents are still talking about that day. The administrator said no one had done something like this before. It made my wife feel like a queen for a day.

My wife will be my love forever. I can't imagine the day she will not say to me, "Hi, hon."

Ed Shaw
Ontario, Canada

But Of Course . . .

As I walk out to the mailbox, I fantasize that I will open the flap and inside I will find an envelope from Lois, addressed to me in her midwestern schoolmistress handwriting. Another Lois Letter to read and cherish.

For twenty-five years our letters went back and forth between Palos Verdes and San Bernardino in California. Hundreds of those letters are now boxed away in my storage closet. Good times—bad times—whatever we were going through—we felt safe with one another as we emptied our hearts on paper. Phone calls were frequent. Visits to each other's homes were joyful reunions. Our husbands and families became friends, enlarging the circle of our love.

My mailbox has yielded no Lois Letters for the last five years. The Lois I loved, and still love, can no longer write, read, nor recognize me as she lives out her remaining years in an excellent Alzheimer's nursing facility in Pomona. From time to time over our twenty-five years together we had talked about our last years, how we would be there for each other no matter what.

Many of us today are knowledgeable about Alzheimer's disease, especially as the result of learning about the affliction of former president Ronald Reagan. Reading about or seeing stories concerning Alzheimer's on TV is becoming commonplace.

Yet, when someone we know or love is diagnosed with Alzheimer's or some form of dementia, we are in a different place of understanding. What was formerly someone else's story now takes on an immediate, poignant reality. It is no longer about *them*. It is about *us*. We enter entirely new worlds—painful, grief-filled, sad—yet at times incredibly beautiful.

"Incredibly *beautiful?*" you ask. How can it be *beautiful* to sit next to a Lois whom no longer bears even a slight resemblance to that other magnificent woman I have known for thirty years? *Beautiful* when we two can no longer share the music we love, can no longer stay up past midnight discussing our busy lives—groups we belonged to, favorite books and articles—sending each other crazy cartoons? *Beautiful* when we can no longer say good-bye with "I'll write when I get home?" But, I can easily say *beautiful* about my Lois, now a total stranger. I sense *beautiful*, remembering Bob Hope's "Thanks for the Memories."

When I am at the nursing home with Lois; however, I refuse to dwell on those memories. What I choose to remember is the best lesson she ever taught me. Sitting with her in the visitor's room or walking with her endlessly through the halls, I remember most vividly that one phrase she gave me years ago. I whisper silently, "But of course . . ."

That particular phrase became one of the favorite mantras we used so many times. *B.O.C.* When I would puzzle about a certain problem, Lois never offered me the answer. Gently, she would turn that problem back to me, questioning me, deeper and deeper. Eventually, after stumbling around, I would find the answer on my own. Only then would she grin at me with that delightful mischievous twinkle in her eyes. She would say, "But of course . . ." By refusing to do my homework for me she showed me that I knew the answer all the time. She had nothing to do with it.

B.O.C.—we are fully alive only in the moment, she would tell me. She didn't imply that we should disregard our past.

We could learn from it best by living fully in the present. We accept what *is*—right now. When we can say "but of course" to life, we don't need to resist or try to control the present. Our B.O.C. mantra was our finest gift to each other.

On one of my recent visits to her, she reached out to greet and hug me, telling me with that same wonderful grin, "You know–you look just like someone I know, but I can't remember her name!" Hugging her back, I reassured her that I was indeed the very person she still knows. I told her my name, which she repeated with "But of course . . ." I knew she would forget my name the next instant.

We had a great visit, being with her just as she was in the moment, chatting away, with our conversation making no or little sense. Neither of us minded much. I didn't care whether or not she remembered me then or would even remember that we had visited with one another. It was "but of course" time for us . . .

These days when I visit her or whenever I think about her, I experience not one but two Loises—the woman who doesn't know my name when I greet her, but who is obviously so delighted just to see and hug me—and within that same physical body, the other Lois, whose bright spirit is almost palpable, overwhelming me by her beautiful soul, her unending love, her irrepressible joy. I am with these two women at all times. I love them both.

Yes, Alzheimer's has cruelly claimed her mind. I leave the nursing home after our last hugs and kisses. Driving home, I take with me my own Lois, who remains always gloriously alive.

But of course . . .

Phyllis Major
Palm Desert, California

SECTION FIVE

NEARING LIFE'S ULTIMATE TRANSITION

*A*s our loved ones enter life's eleventh hour and prepare to take the ultimate journey—passing from this life to whatever lies beyond—each of us deals uniquely with this upcoming separation. For some, the pain of letting go is unbearable. For others, this is not a loss of life; rather our loved ones are given the freedom to take the next step—one without pain and the demented agony of mindlessness. Some of us try to view this transition as a celebration of life.

Hospice workers and other caregivers who work with people during their final months, weeks, and hours are some of the most enlightened and special people in this world. At a patient's bedside these people see life stripped away from all of its pretenses and facades. They learn the essence of what life is during someone's final hours. These caregivers are special because they have a gift for helping people during this transition. In our world, where the focus is on youth and living, it is hard to develop a relationship with someone who will soon die. What a gift—to learn what LIFE means from someone who has only days or weeks to live.

After my father had lived in a nursing home for several years, his health began to decline so much that I inquired about hospice care. Everyone agreed that it was too early. Still, my husband and I anticipated *that* phone call. We learned to make the most of my father's and our time together. And then it happened one evening; quite suddenly. My father suffered a massive stroke. The staff was right there, but despite their efforts to revive him, within thirty minutes he was gone. He wanted it that way. Quick. I had always wanted to be by his side as he passed on, yet this was not to be.

I think about friends and family who have passed on. I've

come to believe that during the last hours of life with a terminal disease, people can choose when they want to go (except for those who die suddenly). Perhaps this is why we hear stories about family members holding vigil for hours at one's bedside; and during those few moments when they leave to get a cup of coffee, their loved one passes on.

Then there are those who manage to share this transition with their loved one—comforting them, holding hands, praying, singing, and sharing sweet memories.

Whether we are at our loved one's side as they take life's ultimate transition or whether they do it without us, we are each granted one gift—a lifetime of memories. We conclude this book with a selection of caregivers' remembrances of times before, during, and after their loved one's ultimate transition that will warm your heart—a true celebration of LIFE.

Perfect In Every Way

I became a member of the Heartwarmers online community about a year ago. I read the stories and felt the warmth of these people, but not with as much dedication and enthusiasm as I had expected. It took a series of little coincidences to help me more deeply understand and be inspired to write and make my small contribution. I admit, I am not a writer nor do I consider myself an educated individual.

This past week has been difficult—we lost our mother. Though not entirely unexpected, it came too quickly, and without warning. There was no time to do those things that help heal the heart and put the mind at ease during a distressing time. Yet, we managed.

I even received a small miracle.

I have felt the love and caring of many people. Most, like those in the Heartwarmers community, I do not even know. I believe I am now on a road to true fulfillment, and Heartwarmers is one of the signposts along the way. I finally *feel* the words. I don't just *read* them.

⁂ ⁂

Mom had a trying life, born one of four daughters of a fur trapper in northern Ontario. The nearest community was only an occasional stop on the rail line, and with the demise of the fur trade, it disappeared long ago. Strife was no stranger to my mother's family. They lost their mother when they were children. Unable to care for his young in the harsh north, my grandfather took his girls to a convent, where my mother's oldest and youngest siblings passed away.

After a time, my mother became ill and had to be sent to Toronto for surgery. Last rites were performed and she was not expected to make it. She did, however, live; and she went on to meet and marry my father. After eighteen years of true love, he passed away.

Of all the trials before and after, this was the harshest. Yet, Mom carried on as best she could, and taught my sister and me much about strength and perseverance. She tried to teach us about love and caring, but we were so angry at the cruelties of the world, we did not see—until this past week.

※ ※

In December Mom was diagnosed with both Alzheimer's and breast cancer. A mastectomy had to be performed. Confused and scared, she looked to me to take care of her. I did the best I could. We grew closer than we had before, and she recovered wonderfully. After a battery of tests the prognosis was that the cancer had not spread, yet there was still a chance it would within one to five years. She was now in a staffed facility because of the Alzheimer's.

Without warning, Mom became ill. On Tuesday they sent her to the hospital, suspecting the flu or a bladder infection. By Thursday she was gone.

Unbeknownst to me, she had prepared for that fateful day. I found out that every detail was predetermined—pall bearers, flowers, casket, who would receive her cross, who would read the prayers—everything.

The only thing was the eulogy. I didn't feel I could do it. No one or nothing was forthcoming. On the night before the service, I serenely admitted to myself it would have to be me. I was unprepared. To find the words I began searching the Web. Effortlessly, exactly what I needed came to me.

I forgot to inform the funeral director of the change until we were entering the church. Horrified, she said there was no way to let the priest know at this point. Yet I was enveloped by a surreal confidence that everything would work out. My sister said there were many good people thinking about us, and to draw on the strength of their thoughts and feelings. I actually felt it. I would like to think that the inner goodness of people like my fellow Heartwarmers helped. Through a fog I delivered, according to others, a fitting and moving tribute to my mother.

My miracle?

In my yard is a rosebush I planted in memory of my dear golden retriever. My mother and my dog had loved each other very much. I wanted a rose to place with my mother, as comfort and a gesture of my love. My wife thought the same thing, and came back from the yard with the disappointing news that all the flowers were wilted and old; there were no new buds.

On the morning of the service, after staying up most of the night writing the eulogy, I was feeling the strength of many heartfelt wishes. I went out to the rosebush myself, wishing for one single rose.

And there it was. Perfect in every way. Just like love.

Carl Sonego
Brooklin, Ontario, Canada

(Editor's Note: Heartwarmers offers inspiration each morning. For information see http://www.heartwarmers.com or to receive a free online subscription, send an e-mail to: join@heartwarmers.com)

That's My Baby!

My mom had a hard life. She was married six times. Her last husband died in 1974. As a widow she did okay. Married or not, Ma was known as a hell-raiser, an independent woman who spoke her mind. She could hold her own with any truck driver!

On October 11, 1996, I got the call no child wants to receive. Ma was being taken by ambulance to the hospital. When I arrived at the hospital they told me she had suffered a stroke. She knew me, and for that I was very glad. Things, however, went downhill from there.

Ma thought she was in Los Angeles. She thought her cousin had left her at the hospital with her brother, with whom Ma hadn't spoken in over twenty-five years (both had passed away).

The doctors used the word *dementia*. They said that Ma's condition would not improve. I was worried, but thought Ma would overcome this, as she always did when facing difficult times. Oops! This was my first wrong thought!

They moved Ma to the interim care part of the hospital. I wondered what that meant. It was a place for Ma to improve a bit so she could be admitted into the rehab part of the hospital, where I first started to figure out the humor, and yes, the joys, of dementia!

The physical therapist at the interim care unit told me that Ma had done okay on the parallel bars! GREAT! When I went into her room, I asked Ma how her day was and what she had done. Ma said she had done nothing! I told her I had heard she had done well at the bars. Ma exclaimed, "BARS? I haven't been to the bars!"

I arrived at the interim care unit on another afternoon when her favorite soap opera was on. The television wasn't on. I asked Ma, "Why aren't you watching your soap opera?"

She retorts, "Hell, I am living in a soap opera."

The time came when Ma had to move out of the interim part of the hospital. We had forty-eight hours to place her. After doing many interviews, I made the decision to place Ma at LaCrosse Rehabilitation Center. This decision was partly based on the physical therapist at the Center, a guy that I thought Mom would do well with. (She loves her guys!)

The stay at LaCrosse was short. Ma fell six times in four months! Those phone calls were so hard. I got the bright idea to bring Ma home. I broached the idea to my husband, telling him to have a stiff drink while he listened. We agreed to bring Ma home. As we were pulling away from the facility, my husband said these words, "This day will go down in infamy!"

Many well-intentioned, good friends even made side bets. "This will never last six months!" I was determined to prove them wrong!

I had done my homework and discovered there were community services, such as adult day care. I enrolled Ma. On the first day, June 25, 1997, the van picked her up and I felt like my child was going away on the first day of school! Day care ended up being my lifeline! At first Ma called it *work*, but soon it was called *school*. Ma would always giggle when we mentioned *school*.

And then, it happened on November 20, 2000. Ma had not said much for about a year and half. Typically my husband, Leo, would care for Ma on Mondays after she got home from *school*. Leo was helping her get settled for an afternoon nap.

He came upstairs and asked me for help. I said, "Sure" and went downstairs to help him. Leo already had Ma on the bed. I rounded the corner of the bed and Ma, with emotion and recognition in her eyes, exclaimed, "THAT'S MY BABY!" I cried! I told Ma it was the best birthday present I had received, as the next day was my forty-eighth birthday.

When I went downstairs to help Ma get ready the next morning, I asked her what she had been doing forty-eight years ago. Sadly, no words came. Her declaration from the night before would be the last words I heard from her, but the *high* of hearing those words carried me through lots of hard times to come.

When I think back, I felt joy at being able to care for my mother until she passed in her sleep on March 13, 2001. Even to this day I can't help but smile when I think of those three little words.

Mary Gilley-Tracy
Spokane, Washington

Do You Know Something?

On November 29, 2000, my dear father, Gerald Hansen, took up his heavenly residence. In addition to other health problems, he had Alzheimer's disease for many years. During his final days, Dad was unresponsive. He had a fixed stare, his eyes did not blink, and he never turned his head; yet he gave us a very special gift in his final moments.

We knew he was dying and had been at his bedside for several hours when the nurses asked that we step out so they could clean him. It was impossible not to notice when we came back into the room that Dad had his head turned differently and was gazing up into the corner over his left shoulder. I told my sister that he would be leaving us very soon, that perhaps his fixation was on an angel coming to usher him home. "I'm But a Stranger Here, Heaven is My Home" had always been one of his favorite songs.

Immediately after I whispered this to my sister, my father moved his head. One by one he deliberately looked into the faces of each of his children and his wife, rotating his head around the bed. When he had finished, and we had each told him how much we loved him, he gazed back up into the corner with a peaceful stare and was gone.

Just before Christmas I returned to the nursing home with gifts my sister and I had prepared for the staff. I dropped them off at the front desk with a cheery "Merry Christmas," even though I wasn't feeling too merry. I did not go onto the Alzheimer's unit, where my father had been the last two weeks of his life. Up until that time my mother had cared for Dad in their home. I just was not ready to get that close to those memories.

The visit lasted only a few minutes. At least I accomplished what I needed to do.

Three weeks ago I needed to return to the nursing home for a meeting to prepare for the Alzheimer's Association's Annual Memory Walk. I was uncertain where to go and asked for directions. It was up on the unit where my father had passed away. *Oh, great!* I thought, dreading the return, despite Dad's lovely, final good-bye.

When I got up on the floor I did not see the group and asked again where to go. Immediately, I recognized one of the nurses who was with Dad at the end. She smiled instantly and said, "I know you. You're Mr. Hansen's daughter." This was almost seven months ago, I thought, and Dad was only here two weeks. I was amazed that she remembered. There was great comfort in her recognition and remembrance. I was moved and fought tears.

Before heading back to the lower level, where the meeting was being held, and as I waited for the elevator, an elderly resident approached me and asked, "Do you know something?"

I smiled and told her that I hoped so. "Well, I don't know *nothing*!" she replied adamantly. It was hard not to be amused.

Fearful that the elevator door would open at any second and I would have to keep her from getting on, I was relieved to spot another elderly woman walking down the hall. When the resident asked again if I knew anything I suggested that maybe the lady walking down the hall knew something.

She looked down the hall at the woman and shouted as she tried to catch up to her, "Do you know something? I don't know *nothing*!"

At the same time a spry little woman with a walker came

out of another room and said, "She's right! She knows nothing! Morning, noon, and night she knows *nothing*! It doesn't matter who knows something. She knows *nothing*! She's right."

I suggested that maybe she could help the woman. But she confessed that they all needed all the help they could get and that she wondered sometimes if God even realized that. I smiled and assured her that I thought He did. She winked and gave me the slyest smile. Her response was, "*You* know something."

With that, the elevator opened and I waved good-bye. As I rode down I could not help but think of my dear friend Brenda's book on finding the joy. I hadn't been able to do so before that moment or to make myself read the book, though I had read a couple of excerpts from a small promotional booklet released before the book's publication. I think I knew Brenda was right, but I just was not ready. I still missed my dad too much.

Now, I know. It is not impossible to find the joy. I thank Brenda for prompting me to look and for modeling that message to us all despite the skeptics.

Brenda, you knew something, I sure didn't!

Jill Wilson
Racine, Wisconsin

Why I Go Back

After my father made life's ultimate transition in March 2001, I returned to the Antelope Valley Care Center (AVCC) where he lived his final years.

Initially, family members were surprised to see me. Oftentimes when a resident dies, surviving family members find it difficult to return. I imagine this is especially difficult for spouses, and even *parents*, of loved ones who have passed on.

Yet, how could I stay away? The residents of this 200-bed Alzheimer's facility and their family members became part of my family while my father was alive. I learned about some of their families and sometimes even about their family history. Although my father was no longer living, they were still alive. They helped me feel connected and feel like I had not lost everything. They enjoy seeing me and I enjoy visiting them.

So, I continue to visit. If someone has a need, I bring it to the nurse's or aide's attention. And then, just as I did for my father, I follow up with the staff to make sure the problem is taken care of. Family members initially wondered if I was becoming a "patient advocate."

Actually, I just wanted to make sure all of my *babies*, as I affectionately call them, were being taken care of. A few staff members knew when I'd ask, "How are all my babies?" They'd smile and, name by name, tell me how each was doing. Then I'd visit everyone I knew and sometimes meet their new roommates. My *family* grew. When one died, a part of me went with him or her. Sometimes I was shocked when I learned of one's passing because s/he had been doing surprisingly well. Other times I knew it could be only a matter of months, weeks, or sometimes days.

This is where I received firsthand knowledge of the value of each day, because LIFE is so fragile.

There are quite a few who have impacted my life in one way or another. I will write about four of them here.

❋ ❋

Rita suffered from crippling rheumatoid arthritis. In her eighties, she was alert and used a wheelchair. Each time I'd visit she was happy to see me. We'd hug and exchange kisses. Rita lost her husband five months after my father died.

When I spent time with Rita, I often wondered what life would be like as I aged, since David and I did not have children either. She was a sweet lady who could still express herself despite the ravages of dementia, and we had fun.

I'd push her in her wheelchair, and on two occasions we raced in the hall toward the dining room. She'd giggle. Of course, just as we reached the end of the hall both times, a different staff member caught us. Despite our combined age exceeding 120 years, we cowered like children in big trouble when the staff members gave us cautionary looks of warning.

While in the dining room, I'd help Rita eat and help her drink her coffee or supplement. She could hold her own cup, but it was easier for her if I reached for it and handed it to her and then took it after she had a drink. I gave her the opportunity to do as much as she could for herself, but some days her arthritis was so painful that the little things meant a lot, like cutting up her food and placing bite-sized pieces on her fork or scooping up a spoonful of JELL-O® gelatin or pudding for her to eat.

Rita was having a harder time hearing. I'd have to lean

forward and speak into her left ear so she could hear me. But even her good ear did not function very well. She'd repeatedly ask, "What? Huh?" Eventually, I asked the nursing staff to check her ears for obstruction and to contact her family.

I always looked forward to my visits with Rita. Especially since she often was the first person I'd see when I walked through the front door. Sadly, Rita passed away a few months later.

❋ ❋

There is Don, whose wife, Marion, is actively involved with his care. She visits and volunteers at the nursing home regularly. She received the Volunteer of the Year Award in 2002. I think Don's smile and the way he acts is so endearing. (A photo of he and Marion appears in the first volume of *Finding the JOY in Alzheimer's*.)

Don was a handsome man. Yet after repeatedly losing his dentures, the staff stopped putting them in his mouth. Over time, his lips adjusted by shrinking around his gums. I am saddened to see him aging so visibly. While he was able to walk, I'd approach him and say something sweet and then smile. He had no idea what I said, but his eyes would look into mine and gleam, and then his face would break out into a big smile.

One day while Marion was visiting him, she turned to talk with a fellow caregiver and when she returned her attention to Don, he was no longer there. She stood to look around and spotted him walking down the hall, hand-in- hand with another woman! All she could do was laugh.

These days, Don's Alzheimer's has progressed so much that he no longer walks. He spends most of his time in a Geri chair. Most often his attention is elsewhere. In the rare moments I am able to capture his attention, lines slowly extend from the corners of his eyes as his toothless smile shadows the man he once was. I still say silly things to him and watch his face closely, knowing his brain struggles to make sense of who I am and what I'm saying.

⁂ ⁂

My sweet Edith. She and my father, both using wheelchairs, would share a table in a special assisted-feeding room—the staff would help them feed themselves. I helped my father eat his food if I visited during mealtimes. We tried to make it a fun experience. Edith would watch me quietly. When my father would spill food on himself and I rushed to get extra napkins, Edith watched. When my father grabbed his drink, sucked liquid through the straw while tilting the plastic cup too far and it poured down his chest, Edith watched. When my father grabbed uneaten food off Edith's tray, Edith calmly watched. She watched as if she were being entertained. I assumed she enjoyed watching us.

Once, I asked her if we were providing entertainment and her face broke into a smile. Sometimes I'd help her with her food—move her drink closer to her, open her milk carton, but she always fed herself. When she was tired and wanted to go *home*, I'd wheel her to her room, or ask my husband, David, or a staff member, to take her *home*. This seemed to be her routine when we visited. Right after dinner, she would go to her room and get ready for bed.

One night after dinner, I asked Edith how many children she had. She said, "Twelve." I did not believe her. I asked a staff member. She said she did not know because she was new. She added that she doubted it, because Edith tells her different things. That evening after dinner I wheeled Edith back to her room and finally noticed the proof of her amazing legacy. Above her bed was an embroidered celebration of her eighty-fourth birthday and her family. The month and the year were embroidered, along with the number of children—twelve, and the number of grandchildren, great-grandchildren and even great great grandchildren!

WOW! I was humbled when I realize my husband and I had two cats and only five godchildren.

Lately Edith's health has declined significantly. She spends a lot of time in bed or uses a Geri chair. She is still alert and we continue to enjoy conversation, teasing, and laughter. These days, if she's sleeping, I gently nudge her and she wakes up instantly. She is surprised to see me. Yet, I know the day will come when she will take her ultimate life journey and then I will only have memories. Until then I visit her as often as I can and ask about her when I'm out of town.

✻ ✻

Finally, there's Myron. Myron became my father's roommate when he was admitted to the AVCC. We enjoyed him immensely as he reminded us so much of my father. Myron runs the place. The staff members cringe when I jokingly say this, because Myron *actually tries to run the place*! He keeps a notepad and pens and pencils in his pocket so he can record information, appointments, and take notes. He also colors and draws and is quite proud of his creations, which he enthusiastically shares with me.

Myron used to walk the halls frequently. Tall, purposeful, wearing glasses and a baseball hat, he supervised everything he saw. I'd greet him and ask if he was holding down the fort and making sure everyone was keeping busy. He'd laugh and say, "Yes." Sometimes he'd sit with two other male residents on one of the chairs lining the hallway or he and another male resident would sit on either side of a female resident. I'd approach and he would smile and extend his hand. I teased him with mischievous questions, "Hey, Myron, are you guys up to no good?" "Myron, are you guys keeping an eye on her?" The other residents would usually look up and either smile, laugh, or say something.

Sadly, as this disease does, it takes a little away from Myron each day. These days Myron sits on one of the chairs alone, his head is lowered, and he naps. Sometimes, if it feels right, I will gently wake him and he looks surprised at first and then he gives me a big smile.

※ ※

Why do I return to AVCC? I go back for Myron, Edith, Don, Rita, and the others I have not mentioned. I realize what my *babies* have taught me. They have taught me the value of each day, because LIFE is fragile and that today might be the last time I see them. I will miss them. But they will be with me in my memories.

Brenda Avadian, M.A.
Lancaster, California

Why Does Mother Live?

"Why does God keep your mother alive?" a friend asked when she realized my mother didn't recognize me during a visit to the nursing home. "I can't understand why God keeps people alive when they're no longer useful."

I didn't take offense because I knew my friend didn't understand. She saw only the shell of a woman who had once been a capable, vibrant person. She didn't understand that caring for Mother amidst her challenges with Alzheimer's added a new dimension to my life.

⁂ ⁂

Today, as I delivered the final papers to the probate court to settle Mother's estate and bring her affairs to a close, I reflected upon how much she had brought to my life, without her even knowing it.

I used to watch my grandchildren visit her in the nursing home. They laughed when she chattered to them.

"Grandma, talk to me," the five-year-old insisted and babbled to her until Mother smiled.

"Why do you visit Great Grandma when she doesn't know you?" someone asked my seven-year old granddaughter.

"Because it makes her happy," Kara replied.

These visits played an important role in the children's lives. They accepted her as she was and never wondered why God kept her alive. They only knew they enjoyed their visits and she meant a great deal to our family.

"Your mother has such a wonderful smile," the nursing home staff remarked. "If I'm having a hard day, I stop by her room. She always has a smile for anyone of us who talks to her."

Yet again, in spite of her Alzheimer's, Mother brought joy into others' lives. Caring for her enriched my life. I realized the truth in the Biblical references to the rewards of compassion for others. I learned about my heritage when she peopled our lives with friends and family and stories she pulled from the past. Occasionally she thought I was one of those ancestors, so then I became a part of that past with her. I learned patience as I slowed my steps to hers and tried to understand her world. I learned humor as we laughed over things we couldn't change.

"We don't laugh enough," Mother remarked. I realized laughter rather than scolding was important to our relationship. I learned the deeper love that comes from caring for someone. And I've tried to fill the hole that was made in my life when she died with appreciation for all that Mother taught me during those Alzheimer's years.

⁕ ⁕

After I turn in the final papers to the Probate Registry Office and my daughter, grandson, and I walk out into the sunshine of an autumn day, I remember how much Mother enjoyed this time of year and am determined to keep her memory alive. We reminisce about Mother on our way home and know we wouldn't have these memories if God hadn't kept her alive beyond what many considered her years of usefulness.

Mary Emma Allen
Plymouth, New Hampshire

My Grandfather

I was a grandchild thrice blessed with grandparents who lived to the ripe old ages of 87, 95, and 103. There aren't too many people in their thirties and forties who can boast about having a grandparent, and I still had three. My special love for them and theirs for me caused me to know at the age of eighteen that I wanted to pursue a social work career caring for the elderly.

The grandparent with whom I had a very close relationship was my Pop Pop Alemi, a natural born teaser who made me feel special because I was the one he joked with the most. We had nicknames for each other that no one else knew the origins of, and we used them freely when we were together and in letters when we lived several states apart.

About five years before his death, Pop Pop began to show signs of dementia and slowly progressed in his forgetfulness and increasing need for care. Luckily for us, though, he remained as sweet and easy-going as ever despite his disease. During a family gathering celebrating my mother's sixtieth birthday, we were reminded again of the helpful, gentle soul he still was.

My husband and I had traveled many hours to be there for this special surprise for my mother, and the turnout of friends and family at her home was overwhelming. As the guests arrived, we would carry their coats upstairs and lay them on the bed until there were 100 or more piled ever so carefully atop the twin bed in my old bedroom. As was his custom of late, my grandfather wanted to retire early and, despite the fact that the party was still in full force, we suggested he go upstairs to my parents' room to rest.

During other visits, he would often travel up and down the stairs, asking to go home rather than rest in his daughter's house, but this time it seemed he must have settled very quickly and we all went back to enjoying the celebration. About forty-five minutes later, who should come down the stairs into the center of the party, dressed only in his long johns, but my grandfather. He looked at me and in a very tired voice queried, "Lorie, I hung up all the coats for you. Can I go to bed now?"

Several years later, as he lay gravely ill in the hospital, I went to see him and whispered the words of his favorite song "Winchester Cathedral" ever so softly in his ear. "Winchester Cathedral, you're bringing me down. You stood and you watched as, my baby left town."

Much to my surprise, he whistled back his favorite song.

What a special memory he gave me, especially since he died the very next day.

Lorie Benovic
Bryn Mawr, Pennsylvania

Happy Heavenly Birthday, Mom!

(Editor's Note: Two years before she wrote the following letter to her mom, Debbie sent fellow caregivers this e-mail.)

My sister, Sandee, is visiting from Minnesota, and is staying with Mom. Today she said that she and Mom had a long and very emotional talk about Mom's funeral wishes. Sandee said she has no clue how they ended up on this subject, but that Mom has very definite ideas of what should happen, what music should be played, etc. Sandee, who was taking notes, asked Mom what she wanted to wear. With no hesitation, Mom said, "Oh, you'd better make it shorts . . . it might be HOT where I'm going!"

Thank you Mom, for helping us get through the worst time in our lives and drying our tears with laughter!

November 24, 2001

Dear Mom,

It's so hard to believe that your awful journey into the clutches of dementia is finally over. You've battled this sickening disease for five-and-a-half years now. None of us could understand why you'd been hanging on for so long, when your body had long since completely betrayed you. There had to be some reason. We were always told, "She's hanging on for something! We may never know what it is," they explained; "then again, you may be lucky enough to have it become crystal clear!"

In August 2001, five years after your first of many strokes, Sandee and I finally completed the overwhelming task of cleaning out thirty-two-plus years of "stuff" which had been collected in your house. How does anyone sort through thirty-two years of someone's belongings, deciding what to save, what to pitch, and what to donate to charity? Would we accidentally throw out something important? How will we ever complete this task?

For five days in a row, we held a yard sale, the view of which was partially obstructed by the twenty-five-foot dumpster we rented for quick disposal of the mounds of trash, ruined furniture, and other items that could no longer serve any recognizable purpose, but were saved because of the grip dementia had on your once brilliant mind.

After the fifth day, we still had much of the yard covered with your belongings, even though we offered each item for only five cents, hoping someone would find something they could use and not feel that financial restrictions would keep them from taking it home.

We sadly threw much of it into the dumpster, and bagged up what we thought should be donated to Goodwill. The job was finally done.

Meanwhile, your decline in health was now advancing so quickly, we just begged God each day to take you home, to reunite you with Dad, who went to Heaven twenty-five years ago. You and I even prayed aloud together a month ago, pleading that God would finally free you from the body that trapped you in misery here on Earth.

Still, you hung on, day-by-day, no longer able to see, no longer willing to eat anything but ice cream. At times you were even unable to remember those of us who spent our lives loving you. Why were you hanging on, Mom? Was there someone who hadn't given you permission to go? Was there a lesson you still needed to teach us? Some sort of unfinished business, perhaps? We were clueless. Why would our merciful God continue to keep you here on Earth when your life seemed so horrible?

This past week, as we watched you on your deathbed, your breathing became totally mechanical. You no longer had the strength to utter a single word and your eyes rarely peeked open at us. It was absolutely devastating to watch you like this, Mom.

Then it happened! Sandee got a call from her son's new bride. In July, they had purchased your home of thirty-two years. Walking out to the mailbox, she made an incredible discovery. It was a Bible, a worn-out Bible, but not just ANY Bible. This was YOUR Bible, Mom! There were so many Bibles in your house that we ended up donating various religious books to Goodwill, after keeping the ones we wanted in the family. This Bible was very old, its battered edges made it an easy one to overlook, and it was tossed into the donation pile. How could something so worn-out and faded have much value? We tend to feel that way about so many things, don't we, Mom?

Enclosed in the Bible was the following message from the anonymous angel who returned it:

"I bought this Bible at the Goodwill at 70th & Federal. I thought I should bring it here."

No name, no return address, nothing. The Goodwill at 70th & Federal is at least a forty-five-minute drive from your house, Mom! Why would anyone go to that much trouble? They didn't send it through the mail; they drove it all the way to your house and put it in the mailbox! No one saw a thing.

On Thanksgiving, I woke up at 2:47 a.m., very frightened. I couldn't stop worrying about you, Mom. A horrible feeling

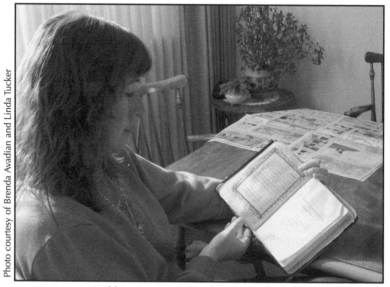

Photo courtesy of Brenda Avadian and Linda Tucker

Debbie Center reading her mother's Bible.

of dread prevented me from sleeping any longer. I finally got out of bed at 4:00 a.m., and went downstairs to prepare a birthday present for a beautiful woman named Millie at the hospice, who I had come to think of as my own angel. She's a resident there, and doesn't understand why God has not yet taken her to Heaven. Her huge smiles and glowing spirit gave me such comfort as I wandered the halls of the hospice, tears streaming down my face as I watched you cling to life.

I went into my living room to check on a tape of music that I was recording for Millie. I was astonished at how orange the room appeared in this beginning of a new day. I looked outside, and the sky was ablaze in God's glory. The sky appeared to be on fire, its stunning gold, yellow, orange, and pink clouds almost hurt my eyes. I knew right then that your day

Debbie Center's mother's Bible.

of release had come, Mom! You always did love a beautiful sunrise or sunset.

A few hours after that sunrise, I arrived at the hospice center. I had received a call on the way there, and a hospice nurse sadly informed me that you were looking really bad, and that if I wanted to see you, I'd better hurry!

I arrived only thirty minutes before Sandee, who had flown in that morning from Minnesota. She was given that Bible by her son when he picked her up at the airport. Sandee brought the Bible to your side, opened it up to the first page she had seen that morning on her way to see you, and read to us the message inscribed on the worn pages, written by YOU, Mom!

You wrote:

"Death to this earthly body is a natural fact, as is birth. To not accept it is to fight nature and to risk one's mind going to pieces. But the real self, the soul, the individual identity of each of us is spirit as is God, and is everlasting, whole, holy, wholesome, vital, change-less as is the love of God. Water, ice, steam, are one and the same but taking different form."

And on another page was written, again in your beautiful pre-dementia handwriting:

"Life After Death," from *Guideposts*, by Norman Vincent Peale—"What is death? Obviously it is a change into some new form of existence. We have allowed ourselves to think of death as a dark door, when actually it is a rainbow bridge spanning the gulf between two worlds. When your body becomes unfit as a dwelling place for your spirit, then it or you will leave the unfit body. But YOU will be more alive than ever before! What a pity to worry about something dreaded that MIGHT happen. If it never happens you've nevertheless ruined otherwise happy days worrying. If it does happen, you're too tired from worry to meet the situation to your best ability."

As we held you close to us, Sandee read this aloud again and again throughout the day, always at your bedside; to all the hospice nurses and grieving loved ones of the other hospice residents. I can't even begin to explain the feelings of peace that YOUR writing gave to all of us preparing to say good-bye to you, Mom! You were so quiet and peaceful, lying there, listening to Sandee repeatedly share your messages with everyone!

Even in your dying hours, you were teaching us the most important lesson you could possibly share with us! You were no longer able to speak with your mouth, but because that angel returned your Bible three months after we'd given it away, and which Sandee and I received the very day of your passing, you spoke to us through the words you'd written in that precious, battered Bible!

Your breathing was reduced to steady puffs of air exhaled through tired lungs, every three seconds. Your beautiful hands that took such loving care of us were now a deep purplish gray in color. Your heart could now only pump blood into your vital organs, so your extremities were very cool and discolored. It is the surest sign that death is only hours away.

I clung so tightly to those purple hands, Mom. My hands looked so pink in contrast to your hands that were deprived of blood flow, and yet yours were actually warmer than my own hands, frozen in the shocking reality that you would be leaving us soon.

There were seven of us in the room with you when you took your final breath on that Thanksgiving Day, November 22, 2001. All three of your children were there, as was your twin sister, one grandson, his new bride, and your daughter-in-law. During the last five minutes of your life, your breathing suddenly changed drastically. No longer were you breathing heavily in mechanical puffs. You were now breathing quietly.

As we all held you tightly, your eyes suddenly opened. You struggled to say something, but none of us could make it out. I pressed my face against yours, kissed your cool face, looked into your brown eyes, and told you to go see Dad, go see what he's been up to the last twenty-five years, and give him a big hug for all of us.

With that, you took one final sigh of relief, and that was the beginning of your new life! With tears streaming down my face, I looked at our hands clutching one another tightly. I was astonished to see your hand immediately return to its normal color! It seemed so symbolic that the death of that body had returned your hand to its normal appearance, Mom! You were free at last, and we all rejoiced through our own tears over what you must be seeing, yes SEEING, after years of blindness!

Happy heavenly birthday, Mom. We shall never forget the lessons you taught us, especially the lessons you brought to us in your final hours. Thank you for hanging on until that angel returned your Bible into our hands once again!

With undying love,
Debbie

Debbie Center
Littleton, Colorado

Five Tips for Caregivers

1. **Treat your loved ones as you would want to be treated, especially if you had their disease.** I consider this the most important of these tips. Once I was able to fully visualize and feel how my life would be like living with this disease, my heart grew with compassion. I can look back today and know that I made the right decisions with the information I had at the time. What a sense of relief given how insecure I felt as a caregiver and how much I questioned myself along the way! If you follow this tip, you will find peace knowing you did the best you knew how; even when making the hard decisions, like placing your loved one in a nursing home.

2. **Attend a support group—whether online or in person, or both.** Initially, I fought the idea of attending a support group. I was already starting work at 5:30 a.m. and working most days until 10:00 p.m. With a schedule like this, I didn't need to join people who were whining about their troubles.

   It took me two months to realize I needed help. Hesitatingly, I attended one meeting. I took so many notes that I returned the following week. Eventually, I made time by starting work at 4:30 a.m. I drew strength from being with others who truly understood my challenges and with whom I could laugh.

   With their encouragement I began writing about caregiving and Alzheimer's, starting with *"Where's my shoes?" My Father's Walk Through Alzheimer's.*

If you can't find a support group that suits you, keep looking until you find one that does. For caregivers living in rural areas, online support groups are lifesavers. Mine has become my *LIFE SUPPORT GROUP.*

3. **Know that your loved one may act out—be paranoid, make accusations, strike out, insist on driving, etc.— because s/he is *afraid*.** My father knew he was losing his ability to remember or find the right words to express himself. Afraid of the uncertainty that lay ahead, he acted aggressively, trying to keep in control of his life—one time he even refused to return home. Once I realized that he was afraid I was better able to deal with his behavior, despite not knowing what to expect.

4. **Care for yourself.** As hard as this is to do while walking the caregiving road of uncertainty, exhaustion, grief, frustration, and sleeplessness, caregivers must care for themselves. Start by following the first three tips and then planning a respite. Have a friend, family, church member, or someone from a home-care agency stay with your loved one while you go somewhere for fun. Escape for two days and one night. Sometimes a planned respite every six months gives you strength just by giving you something to look forward to. Anyone who judges you negatively for taking respite in order to better care for your loved one has not walked in the shoes of a caregiver. Know that caregiving martyrs are not heroes. Take care of yourself so you have the strength to care for your loved one.

5. **Find the JOY in Alzheimer's.** The joys can be big or small. Still, they are moments that cause you to smile.

Seek out these moments each day with your loved one, during support group meetings where members share their experiences, and while reviewing this book or reading the first volume of *Finding the JOY in Alzheimer's*. Take another step: consider writing your joyful moments.

Resources

AgeLine
Tel: 202-434-6231 E-mail: ageline@aarp.org
Website: http://research.aarp.org/ageline/home.html
An online searchable database produced and updated regularly
by American Association of Retired Persons (AARP) of sum-
maries of publications about aging, including books, journal and
magazine articles, research reports, and videos.

Alzheimer's Association
225 North Michigan Ave., 17th Flr., Chicago, IL 60601-7633
Tel: 1-800-272-3900 Website: www.Alz.org
The Alzheimer's Association, a national network of chapters, is
the largest national voluntary health organization committed to
finding a cure for Alzheimer's and helping those affected by the
disease. Call for support group information and to find the
chapter nearest you. See below for information on Memories in
the Making™ and the Safe Return Program.

Alzheimer's Disease Education and Referral (ADEAR)
NIA News: Research on Alzheimer's Disease
P.O. Box 8250, Silver Spring, MD 20907-8250
Tel: 1-800-438-4380 E-mail: adear@alzheimers.org
Website: www.alzheimers.org/banners/5.html
Information about Alzheimer's disease and related disorders.
The ADEAR Center is a service of the National Institute on
Aging (NIA).

American Health Assistance Foundation
15825 Shady Grove Road, Suite 140, Rockville, MD 20850
Tel: 1-800-437-2423 Website: www.ahaf.org

Children of Aging Parents (CAPS)
1609 Woodbourne Rd., Suite 302A,
Levittown, PA 19057-1511
Tel: 1-215-945-6900 1-800-227-7294
Website:
www.careguide.net/careguide.cgi/ caps/capshome.html
Information and referrals, network of support groups, publications and programs to promote public awareness of the value and needs of caregivers. Membership fee.

Dementia Advocacy and Support Network International (DASNI)
P.O. Box 1645 Mariposa, California U.S.A. 95338
Website: http://www.dasninternational.org/
DASNI's purpose is to promote respect and dignity for persons with dementia, provide a forum for the exchange of information, encourage support mechanisms such as local groups, counseling, and Internet linkages, and to advocate for services.

Eldercare Locator
Tel: 1-800-677-1116
Tel: 202-296-8130 Website: www.n4a.org
A free nationwide directory assistance service to help older persons and caregivers locate local support resources. Administered through the National Association of Area Agencies on Aging in Washington, D.C.

ElderCare Online—Internet Community of Elder Caregivers
Website: www.ec-online.net/
ElderCare Online's Neighborhood Network contains links to state, county, and local resources, including Alzheimer's disease support groups and Area Agencies on Aging. Website: www.ec-online.net/Community/Neighborhood/neighborhood.html

Family Caregiver Alliance
690 Market Street, Suite 600, San Francisco, CA 94104
Tel: 1-415-434-3388 Website: www.caregiver.org
This website features a clearinghouse of research findings, resources of hands-on information for caregivers, news bureau, interviews with leaders in the field, public policy, and links to helpful sites.

Memories in the Making™
Tel: 714-283-1111
This signature art program of the Alzheimer's Association of Orange County, California, helps improve the quality of life for people suffering from Alzheimer's disease. When words fail, art allows the individual with Alzheimer's another way to communicate feelings.

National Alliance of Caregiving
4720 Montgomery Lane, Suite 642, Bethesda, MD 20814
Tel: 1-301-718-8444 Website: www.caregiving.org
A national resource center on family caregiving—research and national programs to support family caregivers.

National Institute on Aging (NIA)
One of the National Institutes of Health under the U.S. Department of Health and Human Services.
NIA News: Research on Alzheimer's Disease
Website: www.alzheimers.org/nianews/nianews.html

National Family Caregivers Association (NFCA)
10400 Connecticut Avenue, Suite 500, Kensington, MD 20895-3944 Tel: 301-942-6430 1-800-896-3650
E-mail: info@nfcacares.org Website: www.nfcacares.org
The NFCA is a grassroots organization created to educate, support, empower, and speak up for the millions of Americans who

care for chronically ill, aged, or disabled loved ones. Inquire about free membership for family caregivers.

National Organization For Empowering Caregivers (NOFEC)

Website: www.nofec.org

Provides assistance, education, support and referrals for family/informal caregivers, as well as to promote public awareness about the realities of those who care for loved ones. NOFEC umbrellas Empowering Caregivers www.caregivers.com, which provides a wealth of information, articles, emotional and spiritual support, journal exercises, and tools for empowering caregivers and those they care for.

Safe Return Program

The Alzheimer's Association's nationwide program that assists in the identification and safe and timely return of people with Alzheimer's disease and related disorders who wander. See "Alzheimer's Association" for more information.

TheCaregiversVoice.com

P.O. Box 259, Lancaster, CA 93584

Tel: 661-945-7529 Website: www.TheCaregiversVoice.com

Newly launched website to give a voice to the millions of caregivers who quietly provide care for loved ones. Access this site for news updates, links to other informative sites, and to submit your stories for the *Finding the JOY* series of books.

Well Spouse Foundation

30 East 40th Street, PH, New York, NY 10016

Tel: 1-212-685-8815   1-800-838-0879

Website: www.wellspouse.org

Nonprofit organization providing support and information to well partners of the chronically ill and/or disabled. Provides networking, local self-help support groups, bi-monthly newsletter and round-robin letters. Educates professionals and the public about the needs of spousal caregivers. Membership fee.

Suggested Reading/Listening

Allen, Mary Emma. *When We Become the Parent to our Parents*. MEA Productions, 1998.

Avadian, Brenda, M.A., *Finding the JOY in Alzheimer's: Caregivers Share the Joyful Times*. North Star Books, 2002.

Avadian, Brenda, MA. *"Where's my shoes?" My Father's Walk Through Alzheimer's*. North Star Books, 1999. (Also available in Spanish—"¿Dónde están mis zapatos?" and in German—Die Zeit mit dir.)

Avadian, Brenda, M.A. (author) and Barbara Caruso (narrator). *"Where's my shoes?" My Father's Walk Through Alzheimer's*. Unabridged audio book. Recorded Books, LLC, 2000.

Bell, Virginia and David Troxel. *The Best Friends Approach to Alzheimer's Care*. Health Professions Press, 1997.

Brackey, Jolene. *Creating Moments of Joy for the Person with Alzheimer's or Dementia: A Journal for Caregivers*. Purdue University Press, 2000.

Caregiving! monthly print publication (annual subscription $29.95). Tad Publishing Co., P.O. Box 224, Park Ridge, IL 60068. Website: www.caregiving.com Tel: 847-823-0639

Caregiving.com—"Solutions to your Caregiving Situations throughout your Caregiving Years," Tad Publishing Co., P.O. Box 224, Park Ridge, IL 60068. Website: www.caregiving.com

FitzRay, B.J. *Alzheimer's Activities: Hundreds of Activities for Men and Women with Alzheimer's Disease and Related Disorders.* Ravye Productions, 2001.

Hardship into Hope: The Rewards of Caregiving. (Audiocassette). Connie Goldman Productions, 1999. 217 West Canyon Drive, Hudson, WI 54016 Tel: 715-531-0390 E-mail: congoldman@aol.com

Mace, Nancy L., M.A. and Peter V. Rabins, M.D., M.P.H. *The 36-Hour Day: A Family Guide to Caring for Persons with Alzheimer Disease, Related Dementing Illnesses, and Memory Loss in Later Life.* (3rd Edition). Johns Hopkins University Press, 1999.

McLeod, Beth Witrogen, ed. *And Thou Shalt Honor: The Caregiver's Companion.* Rodale, 2002.

Peterson, Ronald, M.D., Ph.D., ed. *Mayo Clinic on Alzheimer's Disease.* Mayo Clinic Health Information, 2002.

Stobbe, Karen, *Sometimes Ya Gotta Laugh: Caregiving, laughter, stress, and Alzheimer's disease.* Published through funding by the Helen Bader Foundation and the Greater Milwaukee Foundation. ©2002 To order copies: monkar@execpc.com or Karen Stobbe 1536 N 48th St., Milwaukee, WI 53208

The Ribbon—free online newsletter for families and caregivers dealing with Alzheimer's disease and other dementias. Subscribe on line at website: www.theribbon.com, or by mail at The Ribbon, 1104A Murfreesboro Pike, PMB 114, Nashville, TN 37217-1918.

Today's Caregiver—the first national magazine dedicated to caregivers. Caregiver Media Group, 6365 Taft Street, Suite 3006, Hollywood, FL 33024. Tel: 954-893-0550 E-mail: info@caregiver.com Website: www.caregiver.com

Contributors' Biographies

Jamie AGUILAR has cared for two grandmothers with Alzheimer's and one grandfather with CHF. She is now caring for her husband and mother who both have dementia and diabetes. Jamie is Co-founder and Co-editor of *The Ribbon*, a newsletter for families and caregivers of people with Alzheimer's and dementia. "Father's Day" ©2002 Jamie Aguilar

Mary Emma ALLEN writes about Alzheimer's for children and adults. She wrote *When We Become the Parent to Our Parents*, chronicling her mother's encounter with this disease, to encourage caregivers. Her stories appear in *Finding the Joy in Alzheimer's, Vol. I*. Mary Emma speaks to groups about Alzheimer's and caregiving. Website: http://homepage.fcgnet works.net/jetent/mea; E-mail: me.allen@juno.com. "A Secret Communication" and "Why Does Mother Live?" ©2002 Mary Emma Allen

ANONYMOUS Despite efforts to find the creators of these works in order to give them credit, we included them here because they bring JOY. "I Have AAADD!" "The Marriage Proposal," "It Pays to go to School," "A Lady's Bequest," "Senility Prayer," "That's MY Car!" "Ladies Out For a Ride," and "Write it Down!"

Lorie BENOVIC is a mother of two teenagers and a daughter of parents who are now eighty and eighty-five. Long life runs in her family. She lives with her scientist husband in Delaware County, Pennsylvania, and has worked for many years with elderly people and their caregivers. "My Grandfather" ©2002 Lorie Benovic

Debbie CENTER lives in Littleton, Colorado, teaching piano and enjoying her family. A caregiver to her late mom, who had Alzheimer's, Debbie's stories are also featured in the first volume of *Finding the JOY in Alzheimer's*. Debbie can be e-mailed at PianoMam@aol. com. "Happy Heavenly Birthday, Mom!" ©2001 Debbie Center

Evelyn DANIEL widow of Donald Daniel, who succumbed to Alzheimer's disease, attended Central State College in Edmond, Oklahoma, and the University of Oklahoma-Norman. Published: *Essays to Myself, Keep Doing it Until You Get it Right, Dialogues with Donald*, and *A Symphony of Mine Own*. "The Neighbor's Bathroom?" ©2002 Evelyn Daniel

Sharon DeMOE lives in Beggs, Oklahoma. One daughter, son-in-law, and four granddaughters are her neighbors. Her youngest daughter, son-in-law, and grandson live a few miles away. Her husband, Jerry, is now in a VA nursing home in Talihina, Oklahoma. Their lives are full and their faith is helping them heal. "Jerry's Dream" ©2001 Sharon DeMoe

Danny and Debbie FISHER reside in Glen Burnie, Maryland with their son, Kevin. Danny operates heavy equipment, while Debbie works part-time as an Independent Kitchen Consultant with The Pampered Chef. "A Young Husband" © 2001 Debbie Fisher "Thank you, GOFers" ©2001 Debbie and Danny Fisher

Mary C. FRIDLEY, RN, BC, is a registered nurse certified in gerontology with more than twenty years in the geriatric health field. She offers caregiver education, consulting, and speaking engagements. Mary is also the author of caregiver advice columns and articles in print and on the World Wide Web. "Superheroes" ©2002 Mary C. Fridley

Heather FROESCHL is the author of thirteen books and hard at work on several more. She is a freelance editor working with numerous authors and publishers. She lives happily in the Blue Ridge Mountains with her family, and way too many pets. Visit her Web page to learn more: www.Quilldipper.com "As Time Goes By" ©2002 Heather Froeschl

Jerry L. GIBSON is currently retired, but had a long career in financial and general management with Exxon Mobil, Riviana Foods, and two other companies that he founded. He earned degrees in accounting and finance from North Texas University and SMU and is a CPA. "To My Wife" ©2002 Jerry L. Gibson

Sallie GIBSON HOLMES, daughter of Gail and Jerry Gibson, was born and raised in Texas. Now living in the Washington D.C. area, she is married and has two terrific children. She is a clinical social worker and an active volunteer in her church and community. "My Mother's Touch" ©2001 Sally Gibson Holmes

Mary GILLEY-TRACY of Spokane, Washington, was in the workforce when she and her husband decided to care for her mother in their home. Mary says, "This day changed our lives. Thanks to all the caregivers we met on the Internet who helped us survive the caregiving challenge." "That's My Baby!" ©2002 Mary Gilley-Tracy

Janice GREENHOUSE lives in Littleton, Colorado with her husband Norman. She adored playing SCRABBLE® with her twin sister Janette Shulman. The whole family is thrilled that she captured on film the typical expression on Janette's face after getting yet another BINGO! "Victory! Janette Shulman of Colorado may show signs of early Alzheimer's, but she hits yet another BINGO by using all seven letters in a game of Scrabble®." ©1996 Janice Greenhouse

Judi HOLTZEN writes "Lynn Keane and her mom are friends and beauty shop clients of mine. Lynn's mom and I have a great time talking and laughing about silly things. To me she is just my friend Charlotte. She can be who she is with me." "Lynn Keane with BUM logo on sweatshirt" Photo ©2001 Judi Holtzen

Faith Bell JACKSON has worked as an activity director, medical social worker, and health care administrator. Her current work is in Bereavement, Volunteers and Spiritual Care for Hospice. Mother of three, grandmother of one, and poet (as f. Hannah) she graduated from Cornell University. "Frannie Bell" ©1999 Faith Bell Jackson

Barbara JACOBSON grew up, married, and raised two boys in Palmdale, California. Upon retirement in 1995, she and her husband became fulltime RV-ers and have been traveling and exploring the USA ever since. Her hobbies are hiking, biking, fishing, birding, writing, photography, and geneal-ogy. "The Power of a Smile" ©2002 Barbara Jacobson

Shirley JENKINS is a widow with two children and two grandchildren. She is a retired elementary school secretary who worked in the Magnolia School District for twenty-nine years. She's lived in her home in Anaheim, California since 1956. "Food Fight by Candlelight" ©2002 Shirley Jenkins

Helen Bennett JONES reminded us to laugh hard and laugh often. She came to each of our support group meetings with a thought-provoking and unconventional question—e.g., *Did Adam and Eve have navels?* She passed away while caring for her husband who followed her a short time later. "Answer the Coffee Cup?" ©1999 Helen Bennett JONES

Lynn S. KEANE writes, "I've been a nurse for twenty-eight years, and continually feel great love from my elderly patients. I live in Colorado; have been married for twenty-two years; and have three beautiful children. I have been writing poetry and short stories since my youth, and my goal is to continue to write and to share my experiences." "Happy Mother's Day" ©2001 Lynn S. Keane

Denise E. KELLEY lives on Cape Cod in Massachusetts. She has been caring for her mother, Dorothy, for six years and operating the family aqua farm with her dad, Olin. Denise writes, "Life leaps from one mini-crisis to the next . . . we deal with each; often in hip boots." "God's Wedding Day Confetti" ©2002 Denise E. Kelley

Linette MADSEN, middle daughter of three, has lovingly taken the caregiving challenge for her parents. The three of them have become one during this journey and Linette believes her parents continue to enrich her life. Her passions also include interior design, photography, gardening, and various crafts whenever she is able to fit them in. "After a successful jump, Loraine Yates is lifted off her feet by Stanley R. Olzaski, Skydive Santa Barbara instructor." Photo ©2002 Linette Madsen

Phyllis MAJOR is a freelance writer. She lives in Palm Desert, California where she contributes to *The Desert Woman*, a Coachella Valley newspaper. She has four sons and four grandchildren. "But of Course . . ." ©2000 Phyllis Major "What Makes Caregiving Rewarding?" ©2001 Phyllis Major

Marion RILEY writes, "I moved to Lancaster, California, from Palmdale, California, to be closer to my husband, Don. He is in a care center for people with Alzheimer's. I visit him often and also volunteer at the center." "Screaming Lady" ©2000 Marion Riley

Ed SHAW writes, "I would like to be known as a little guy from a city in the snow belt of Ontario, Canada, who wanted to tell his story in the hope of helping others deal with this horrible disease. Thank you for allowing it to be told." "My Love, Forever" ©2002 Ed Shaw

Carl SONEGO writes, "A tradesman without a post-secondary education, I was inspired to write this piece from the events surrounding my mother's illness and passing. Though I had never written before, doing so has brought me much peace, serenity, and kind words from many. I hope writing helps others find some comfort too." "Perfect in Every Way" ©2001 Carl Sonego

Marian SUMMERS is caregiver to her husband, Ron, who after several years of home care, is now in The Nebraska Tabitha Health Care Center. They are parents to three children—two daughters: Joyce Hinrichs in Phoenix, Arizona, and Rhonda Jacobs in Long Beach, California; and a son, Richard in Olathe, Kansas. "Those are MY Leaves" ©2002 Marian Summers

Linda TUCKER (PHOTOLJT@sbcglobal.net) resides in Northern California. She is founder of The Gathering Place—Online Alzheimer's Caregiver Support. Linda's father was diagnosed with Alzheimer's in 1997. Linda provides support by continuing to *pay forward* the help she found through Internet chats to those who are just beginning their journey in Alzheimer's. "Did You Ever Dream . . .", "Dreams Do Come True" and photos: "Jamie Aguilar and Karen Bradley, Co-founders of TheRibbon.com"; "Jane's Angels Start the Memory Walk in Nashville, Tennessee ©2001 Linda Tucker

Lorraine H. TUCKER was born in the North Carolina mountains. She writes, "After graduating I left for Virginia's seashore. There I found a job and a husband. Three adorable babies soon followed. Retirement in 1979 found us bound for Texas. Alzheimer's in 1999 found me a caretaker. In 2002 I was a widow." "A Shining Knight" ©2002 Lorraine H. Tucker

Roberta **WERTENBERG** has worked extensively with seniors. Employed by the Riverside County Adult Protective Service's C.A.R.E. Program, Roberta remains passionate about serving Alzheimer's patients and their families. Appointed to the Alzheimer's Advisory Committee for the State of California, Roberta continues to be active in the Alzheimer's Association and Partnership to Preserve Independent Living for Seniors and Persons with Disabilities. "I Developed Hemorrhoids" ©2002 Roberta Wertenberg

Kathy Gade **WHIRITY** is a freelance writer and newspaper columnist. She's been happily married to her husband, Bill, for twenty-six years. With their daughters, Jaime and Katie, away at college, these empty nesters are discovering, with sweet surprise, that the honeymoon isn't over, it's only just begun—again. "A Million Accident-Free Miles"; original title: "Living with Alzheimer's—A Daughter's Point of View" ©2000 Kathy Whirity

Jason **WILLIAMS**, from Northern Illinois, is in the sixth grade. He was ten when he wrote this story. Jason has a twin brother, Jeremy, and a little sister, Jennifer. Jason enjoys sports and playing Nintendo. At the age of six, Jason began helping his Grandpa Dick. He enjoys walking in the Alzheimer's Memory Walk. "A Ten-Year-Old Makes a Difference" ©2002 Jason Williams

Jill M. **WILSON, MS**, is a Geriatric Services Manager of Aurora Health Care—South Region in Wisconsin. "Do You Know Something?" ©2001 Jill M. Wilson

Sharon WRIGHT, Ed.D., MFT is a psychotherapist in Claremont, California. Her favorite topic in giving workshops is "Putting Joy Into Your Life." Formerly Dr. Wright was dean of students at the University of La Verne. Her degrees were earned at Occidental and ULV. She enjoys her stepsons and their families. "Time Stood Still" ©2001 Sharon Wright

Loraine YATES has been caring for her *Little Mama* in her home for the last five years. Loraine writes poetry and short stories about her joyful and challenging life experiences. Besides being a collector of Pepsi® memorabilia, she now has a new hobby—SKYDIVING. "A Caregiver's Prayer" ©2002 Loraine Yates; "Garden of Joy" ©1999 Loraine Yates; "Grounded at 13,500 Feet" ©2002 Loraine Yates

About the Editor

Brenda Avadian, M.A., cared for her ninety-year-old father with Alzheimer's until his passing in 2001. She looks for the humor in life's challenges and is committed to helping fellow caregivers *Find the JOY* when the journey seems impossible.

Avadian, *The Caregivers Voice*, has achieved an international reputation and her books sell around the world. Her passion, enthusiasm, and tireless efforts to help caregivers are why so many organizations invite her to speak about caring for people with Alzheimer's.

Finding the JOY in Alzheimer's: When Tears are Dried with Laughter is her seventh book and follows *Finding the JOY in Alzheimer's: Caregivers Share the JOYFUL Times* and the critically acclaimed *"Where's my shoes?" My Father's Walk Through Alzheimer's*—also available in audio book and in the German (*Die Zeit mit dir*) and Spanish (*"¿Dónde están mis zapatos?"*) languages. Sales proceeds of these books support groups and organizations that help people with Alzheimer's and their families.

Prior to becoming a caregiver, Brenda worked with Lockheed, the International Medical Corps, and the Wisconsin Energy Corporation. She taught at the University of Wisconsin-Milwaukee, Marquette University, Alverno College, and co-designed and facilitated Lockheed's executive development program at the University of Southern California. Her earlier books are about communication competencies, career development, and leadership. She was commissioned a Kentucky Colonel in 1989 for her contributions to public service.

Born in Milwaukee, Wisconsin, Brenda earned her bachelor's and master's degrees from the University of Wisconsin-Milwaukee in 1980 and 1982, respectively. She met her husband, David Borden, in Milwaukee. They now live in Lancaster, California, with their three cats.

Call for Submissions

Have you written a story or poem about a JOYFUL moment caring for your loved one with Alzheimer's?

Do you have a photo or artwork of a JOYFUL activity with your loved one with Alzheimer's?

Dear Caregiver:

I invite you to submit your work for consideration in the third volume of the *Finding the JOY in Alzheimer's* series. Together we will give hope, strength, and courage to caregivers around the world.

The **Criteria** for your JOYful submission are as follows:

Length: 250 to 1,000 words (1 to 4 typed pages double-spaced).

Format: Prefer e-mail. Send as attachment in MSWord. Attach high-resolution digital/scanned photos as .jpg or tif files.

Subjective Criteria: Caregivers should feel JOY when reading your story/poem. Their hearts should fill with hope and JOY when looking at your photo/artwork.

Descriptive Criteria: Your story must contain enough vivid detail so the reader feels s/he is living the experience. Your photo/artwork must capture a JOYful moment.

If your work is accepted, we will include up to a fifty-word biography in the "Contributors' Biographies" section of the book.

Please send your submissions under the subject heading **FtJiA-3** to BrendaAvadian@TheCaregiversVoice.com or mail to Brenda Avadian, TheCaregiversVoice.com, P.O. Box 259, Lancaster, CA 93584.

Together, we will bring hope and JOY to caregivers!

> Genuinely Yours,
> Brenda Avadian, M.A.
> *The Caregiver's Voice*

Order Information

Ask for
Finding the JOY in Alzheimer's ~ 2
When Tears are Dried With Laughter
ISBN 0-9632752-3-2
&

Finding the JOY in Alzheimer's
Caregivers Share the JOYFUL Times
ISBN 0-9632752-2-4

at your neighborhood bookstore or library.

Buy through any online retailer
or
receive a discount and have your purchase support
groups and organizations that help people with
Alzheimer's and their families when you:
Call **Toll FREE 1-800-852-4890**
(Credit Card orders only)
or
Order through our Website
http://www.TheCaregiversVoice.com/books

Also visit our Website for the critically acclaimed
"*Where's my shoes?*"
My Father's Walk Through Alzheimer's
ISBN 0-9632752-1-6

We'd like to hear from you!

Write to the author at:
Brenda Avadian@TheCaregiversVoice.com